Development, Sexual Cultural Practices and HIV/AIDS in Africa

Samantha Page

Development, Sexual Cultural Practices and HIV/AIDS in Africa

palgrave
macmillan

Samantha Page
Department of Global Development
and Planning
University of Adger
Kristiansand, Norway

ISBN 978-3-030-04118-2   ISBN 978-3-030-04119-9 (eBook)
https://doi.org/10.1007/978-3-030-04119-9

Library of Congress Control Number: 2018962020

© The Editor(s) (if applicable) and The Author(s) 2019. This book is an open access publication.
Open Access This book is licensed under the terms of the Creative Commons Attribution 4.0 International License (http://creativecommons.org/licenses/by/4.0/), which permits use, sharing, adaptation, distribution and reproduction in any medium or format, as long as you give appropriate credit to the original author(s) and the source, provide a link to the Creative Commons license and indicate if changes were made.
The images or other third party material in this book are included in the book's Creative Commons license, unless indicated otherwise in a credit line to the material. If material is not included in the book's Creative Commons license and your intended use is not permitted by statutory regulation or exceeds the permitted use, you will need to obtain permission directly from the copyright holder.
The use of general descriptive names, registered names, trademarks, service marks, etc. in this publication does not imply, even in the absence of a specific statement, that such names are exempt from the relevant protective laws and regulations and therefore free for general use.
The publisher, the authors, and the editors are safe to assume that the advice and information in this book are believed to be true and accurate at the date of publication. Neither the publisher nor the authors or the editors give a warranty, express or implied, with respect to the material contained herein or for any errors or omissions that may have been made. The publisher remains neutral with regard to jurisdictional claims in published maps and institutional affiliations.

Cover design by Tom Howey

This Palgrave Macmillan imprint is published by the registered company Springer Nature Switzerland AG
The registered company address is: Gewerbestrasse 11, 6330 Cham, Switzerland

Foreword

Samantha contacted me back in 2008 when she was thinking of doing a Ph.D. about traditional cultural practices and HIV in Malawi. She'd read my research about traditional cultural practices and AIDS.

Initially, Samantha wanted to interview women and girls who had participated in sexual cultural practices. But I said to her perhaps it would be better to interview people who were worked on HIV prevention programmes in Malawi. As an outsider, trying to interview women about a sexual practice shrouded in secrecy is problematic.

Samantha went to Malawi to do her doctoral research in 2008. I met her for the first time there. I employed her to be my research assistant and collect data whilst she was conducting her interviews.

Since then we have been in regular contact and I have provided advice to her on her Ph.D. and her post-doctoral career.

This book is a welcome addition to the dearth of literature on sexual practices and AIDS in Malawi. It is an under researched topic but nevertheless an important one. Many assumptions are made about the link between AIDS and sexual practices so this book is an important contribution to knowledge as it highlights the reality in Malawi, based on 60 interviews with policymakers, programme managers, lawyers and MPs, Malawian and foreign, who work on HIV prevention issues.

What is interesting about her findings is how Malawians volunteer information about sexual cultural practices and AIDS as if they are making themselves appear modern and distancing themselves from the rural villager. Samantha uses the term 'narratives of blame'—I think this is very fitting—in other words how the stories told by Malawians blame the backward villager. In other words, the urban, educated Malawian elite is not responsible for the high HIV prevalence rates in Malawi, rather it is the uneducated, rural person.

Why is this book important? The significant amount of money international donors spend on trying to eradicate or modify sexual cultural practices is unjustified and wrong. So Samantha unravels the story using evidence from her interviews to highlight a flaw in donor thinking. That far too often donors don't use evidence to support their work. They latch on to an idea thinking it is important, when really it isn't.

Los Angeles/Philadelphia, USA   Susan Watkins
Visiting Scholar,
California Center for Population Research,
University of California-Los Angeles,
Professor Emerita of Sociology,
University of Pennsylvania

Acknowledgements

I would like to thank all those I interviewed in Malawi. I would particularly like to thank the family I stayed with in Malawi who were so kind to provide me with accommodation and food and welcomed me to their home. I can't thank you enough.

Thanks to all who supported me at Palgrave Macmillan: Karthika Purushothaman, Alina Yurova and Mary Fata in particular.

Thank you to Tony Chafer. If it wasn't for you I would have dumped the idea of completing a Ph.D. many years ago but you encouraged me to persevere.

I have many mentors. Thank you to Susan Watkins who has provided me with endless support ever since I first became interested in the topic.

A huge thanks also to Louise Ackers. I really appreciate your advice and support.

Thanks to my colleagues in the Faculty of Social Sciences and the library at the University of Agder for providing financial support so that this book can be accessible online.

Also thanks to my colleagues in the Department of Global Development and Planning, especially Hanne Haaland, who gave me the time to write the book, Alf Gunvald Nilsen for pushing me to think about this book, write a proposal and for helping me with the process and reviewing chapters and Gibran Cruz Martinez for reviewing chapters.

Thank you to my wonderful friends Bella and Sandra. Thanks also to Mitty.

Lastly, I owe the deepest of thanks to my Mum and Dad, Martin and Jodie.

Contents

1	Introduction	1
2	Theoretical Perspectives	25
3	The Development Aid Situation in Malawi	43
4	'Harmful Cultural Practices' and AIDS	61
5	How the Church Frames AIDS	107
6	The Construction of Policy: Donors, AIDS and Cultural Practices	141
7	Conclusion and Recommendations	187
	Glossary	199
	Index	203

Abbreviations

AIDS	Acquired Immune Deficiency Syndrome
ATR	African Traditional Religion
CABS	Common Approach to Budgetary Support
CBO	Community Based Organisation
CEDAW	Convention on the Elimination of all forms of Discrimination Against Women
CHAT	Country Harmonisation and Alignment Tool
DFID	Department of International Development
EU	European Union
FBO	Faith-Based Organisation
GBV	Gender Based Violence
GFTAM	Global Fund to fight AIDS, Tuberculosis and Malaria
GTZ	German Technical Development Agency
HADG	HIV/AIDS Development Group
HCP	Harmful Cultural Practice
HIV	Human Immunodeficiency Virus
HMIS	Health Management Information System
IAWP	Integrated Annual Work Plan
INGO	International Non-Governmental Organisation
M&E	Monitoring and Evaluation
MANASO	Malawi Network of AIDS Service Organisations
MANET+	Malawi Network for People Living with HIV/AIDS
MBCA	Malawi Business Coalition on AIDS
MDHS	Malawi Demographic and Health Survey
MDICP	Malawi Diffusion and Ideational Change Project
MGDS	Malawi Growth and Development Strategy

MIAA	Malawi Interfaith AIDS Association
MoE	Ministry of Education
MoH	Ministry of Health
MOWCD	Ministry of Women and Child Development
NAC	National AIDS Commission
NAF	National Action Framework
NAPHAM	National Association for People Living with HIV in Malawi
NGO	Non-Governmental Organisation
NSF	National Strategic Framework
NSO	National Statistical Office
OPC	Office of the President's Cabinet
PEPFAR	The U.S. President's Emergency Plan for AIDS Relief
PLHIV	Persons Living with HIV
PMTCT	Prevention of Mother To Child Transmission
SAFAIDS	Southern Africa HIV/AIDS Information Dissemination Service
STIs	Sexually Transmitted Infections
SWAp	Sector Wide Approach
UNAIDS	Joint United Nations Programme on HIV/AIDS
USG	United States Group
WHO	World Health Organisation

List of Figures

Fig. 1.1 Stop harmful cultural practices banner (Photo taken on 10 July 2009. Malawi: Author) — 2

Fig. 4.1 Difference between global policies on gender-based violence, harmful cultural practices and AIDS and those at the national level (*Source* Author) — 68

Fig. 4.2 HIV prevalence by gender and marital status (% HIV-Positive) among respondents aged 15–24, Malawi (*Source* Watkins [2010] based on data from the Malawi Diffusion and Ideational Change Project [MDICP 2004]) — 85

Fig. 4.3 HIV incidence by gender and age, all ages above age 15, Rural and Urban Malawi, demographic and health survey data, 2005 (*Source* Cited in Watkins [2010] Prepared by Patrick Gerland, United Nations Population Division, from DHS survey data) — 86

Fig. 4.4 HIV incidence by gender and age, all ages above age 15, Rural and Urban, Zambia, demographic and health survey data, 2001–2002 (*Source* Cited in Watkins [2010] Prepared by Patrick Gerland, United Nations Population Division, from DHS survey data) — 87

Fig. 4.5 HIV incidence by gender and age, all ages above age 15, Rural and Urban, Tanzania, demographic and health survey data, 2004–2005 (*Source* Cited in Watkins [2010] Prepared by Patrick Gerland, United Nations Population Division, from DHS survey data) — 88

LIST OF TABLES

Table 4.1	Received information on the following topics at initiation	93
Table 4.2	New knowledge provided during initiation ceremony	94
Table 4.3	List of items liked during initiation ceremonies	95
Table 4.4	List of activities not liked during initiation ceremonies	96
Table 4.5	Negative experiences during the initiation ceremonies by age	97

LIST OF BOXES

Box 6.1	P15 Interview with a District Youth Officer	152
Box 6.2	Response to UNAIDS question	171
Box 6.3	Questions for students on cultural practice and HIV/AIDS	174
Box 6.4	PowerPoint presentation by the Seventh-day Adventist Church	175
Box 6.5	PowerPoint presentation by the Seventh-day Adventist Church Cont	176
Box 6.6	Data from UNAIDS consultancy	176

CHAPTER 1

Introduction

In the mid-1980s, non-governmental organisations (NGOs) began to flow into poor countries to help them improve their lives and livelihoods. Malawi, a small country in south-central Africa, was an attractive location: it is one of the poorest countries in the world, it is peaceful and has little crime, English is the official language, it has reasonable roads such that NGO staff can move around relatively easily. In the period 1985–1989 there were 16 registered NGOs; in 2001–2005 there were 196 NGOs, half of them focused on HIV prevention (Morfit 2011). In the first phase, NGOs typically focused on implementing programmes that would improve health (e.g. clean water) and agriculture. Increasingly, however, they were concerned with improving the situation of women and girls, who were considered to be particularly vulnerable to harms. A hierarchy of NGOs was established. At the top were international NGOs such as Save the Children, Catholic Relief Services and CARE, at the bottom were small organisations based in district capitals.

A major consequence of the establishment of NGOs was that it provided jobs in the formal economy for educated Malawians. Those with a PhD or an MA worked in offices in the Capital, Lilongwe, those with only a BA were stationed in district capitals, and those who had only a secondary education picked up jobs whenever they could, such as working on a short-term survey. The level of education determined not only one's income but also their social status and whether they lived in one of the two large cities or in a district capital. Not surprisingly, those at the

© The Author(s) 2019
S. Page, *Development, Sexual Cultural Practices and HIV/AIDS in Africa*, https://doi.org/10.1007/978-3-030-04119-9_1

top of the income and social status ladder looked down on those who had little or no education.

In 2008, I was working as a Programme Manager for a sexual and reproductive health NGO based in London. As part of my job, I went to Malawi to monitor a HIV prevention programme, funded by the Department for International Development (DfID). I was speaking to a Malawian woman in Blantyre (Malawi's second largest city, located in the South of the country) who set up a Women and AIDS Community Based Organisation (CBO), which was indirectly funded by DfID. She was HIV positive. She spoke English and raised the topic about certain sexual practices said to be risky for the spread of HIV, often referred to in the literature, and by people in Malawi, as 'harmful cultural practices'. One particular practice grabbed my attention. It is called *fisi*), which means 'hyena' in English. The story recounted to me was about a hyena. In this case the hyena is a man, who is hired to have sex with young women who participate in initiation ceremonies when they start menstruating. But the hyena practice has several other meanings, which I will come to later. A few years later, an NGO ran a banner in the daily newspapers—see Fig. 1.1: it was at the bottom of the first page, with a background of red and black, and said 'STOP Harmful cultural practices'. The banner was produced by UNICEF.

I arrived in Lilongwe in 2008 to begin my research and was picked up by my friend who worked for an AIDS NGO. We travelled to Blantyre and she invited me to stay at her house with her family. I asked her if I could work from her office and was fortunate enough to be given desk space.

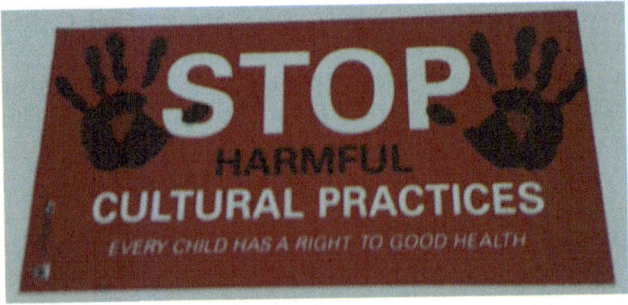

Fig. 1.1 Stop harmful cultural practices banner (Photo taken on 10 July 2009. Malawi: Author)

This was an invaluable opportunity as I shared an office with a policy officer and this enabled me to meet people passing by my desk. I was hoping that I would identify an organisation with which to carry out my research. It was not long after I was in my new surroundings that the Executive Director of a small CBO, based in the district of Mulanje, asked me what I was doing there. He then excitedly told me about the *fisi* practice. He said for him, *fisi* meant three things:

> 1. Surrogacy – if you see a stick on the door you should not go in as you know something is going on. 2. Kuchotsa/kutsatsa fumbi – sexual cleansing. During initiation ceremonies when a girl has reached puberty and is menstruating she is taught how to entertain her husband. The girl could be from 7, 8 or 9-12 years old. She is told she must sleep with someone otherwise she will have problems. The person she will sleep with may be big or young. The impact of this a) early/unwanted pregnancy b) drop out at school c) early marriage d) contract HIV. 3. Kuchotsa milaza – concept whereby in Mulanje you may go out and you have left your husband and you sleep with other men. So you are forced to sleep with someone else who is the relative of the husband to be forgiven for sleeping with someone else. (Journal entry 26 August 2008)

He invited me to visit his village where he ran the CBO to find out more about the *fisi*. However after I visited his village, my friend, the Director of the AIDS NGO, told me that the practice was not particularly prevalent in that part of Malawi, and that he had exaggerated the story so that I would visit and perhaps help him access funding.

So I returned to my desk in Blantyre. Along came the Executive Director of a youth CBO. He told me 'there are lots of cultural practices that go on in my village' and therefore it would be a perfect site to conduct my research. He then described at length the practice of *kusasa fumbi* and then told me:

> When initiation ceremony comes to an end, the village leaders or opinion leaders in the village, they plan for the men to have sex with girls. The men are from a different community. Also women are chosen to have sex with boys. They are also from a different village. Women get women and men get men. They are paid in food. No money. Condoms are not used. There is a need to exchange fluids so cannot use condoms. (Journal entry, 26 August 2008)

I was amazed that they volunteered to tell me about the *fisi* practice without having interviewed them. I then became aware of a widespread misconception in the NGO sector and beyond into the world of international donors that so-called 'harmful cultural practices' were the main driver of the AIDS epidemic in Malawi. It was the educated Malawian elites who described these practices at length, expounding on the risks they presented and efforts to stamp them out, while at the same time weaving into the discourse other fashionable interests of international agencies, such as the particular vulnerability of women, especially young women, to contracting HIV. It is important to highlight here that these stories about harmful cultural practices came from educated Malawians who speak English, not the villagers. But the link between these 'harmful cultural practices' and the epidemic was never supported by evidence. For example, while it is known that the prevalence of AIDS among widows is higher than among married women, there had been—and continues to be—no evidence that this was due to widow inheritance (when a woman's husband dies, she lives with her husband's brother) rather than to years of marriage to a man who had died of AIDS. From a biomedical perspective the latter is more likely.

Biomedical evidence shows that 'harmful cultural practices' are not the main contributors to the AIDS epidemic. So what is interesting is why so many educated Malawians working in the AIDS sector told me about the practices, not the villagers, and blamed them for the spread of AIDS.

In this book I analyse the responses these practices evoke: these include lawyers, researchers, policymakers, government ministers, NGO and INGO staff, staff working for bilateral and multilateral agencies, national and district officials and health workers.

This book explores policy surrounding HIV prevention. It draws attention to the ways that the elites in Malawi—people who stand out because they are educated and thus speak and read English, the official language, in contrast to the majority of Malawians who live in villages and have, at best, completed primary school. Those who have a university degree dominate the policy arena: they are staff in the civil service and they implement the programmes of NGOs and bilateral or multilateral agencies programmes (Watkins and Swidler 2009; Myroniuk 2011). They are middle-class people in government positions or working in International NGOs.

The educated elites I met almost invariably disparage those who have less education. I found that upon meeting an educated Malawian, they often began the conversation by telling me about what came to be called the 'harmful cultural practices' of the uneducated villagers. They thus make it clear to expatriates who buy into the distorted accounts of the elites.

I show that the epistemic community in Malawi (epistemic community includes international donors working on HIV and AIDS as well as the Malawian elite) are reframing both sexual cultural practices and women's rights concepts in the context of what is widely considered an emergency, the AIDS epidemic. This epistemic community comprises those working in the field of AIDS, who frame narratives about AIDS to achieve other goals, both ideal and pragmatic, for example for the purposes of self-preservation and self-interest. Haas' (1992) notion of the 'epistemic community' is particularly useful for conceptualising the HIV prevention community in Malawi. Haas describes an epistemic community as 'a network of professionals with recognised expertise and competence in a particular domain or issue-area' (Haas 1992, p. 3). He says that epistemic communities are groups of professionals, from a variety of different disciplines, which produce policy-relevant knowledge about complex technical issues (Haas 1992, p. 16). This book makes the case that the Malawian elite is influencing the policy agenda on AIDS and harmful cultural practices. This book also examines how others—e.g. international staff working for International NGOs, bi- and multilateral donors—adopted the views provided by the Malawian elite without questioning the evidence. But why would they? First, donors and NGOs have little interest in establishing an evidentiary base for any of their programmes[1] and second, UNAIDS did not want to disseminate the evidence about low probabilities.

I also explore how evidence is produced in the context of AIDS and how certain sexual cultural practices have been co-opted by the NGO discourse in order to explain why HIV prevalence is so high in Malawi as well as other African countries.[2] My analysis is oriented around how different narratives on AIDS are framed, and what and how evidence is used to support them. As I show, these narratives are not based on face-to-face encounters with women involved in these practices. What *is* under consideration is the way the Malawian elites present rural people as backward by deploying the phrase 'harmful cultural practices': the elites then blame the AIDS epidemic on these practices. What my theoretical framework shows is how this constructed and epidemiologically inaccurate narrative has been taken up and endorsed by international donors.

Initially, this research intended to examine the contribution of sexual cultural practices such as widow inheritance and initiation rites (Munthali and Zulu 2007) to the transmission of HIV (Coombes 2001; Chizimba et al. 2004). However, after I read about the exotic cultural practices that are considered harmful (Malawi Human Rights Commission 2006), and the research of epidemiologists (e.g., Gray et al. 2001; Boily et al. 2009) it was apparent that many, perhaps most, of the cultural practices are unlikely to contribute significantly to the epidemic. Far more important are everyday practices, such as unprotected sex with multiple sexual partners both before and after marriage (Smith and Watkins 2005; Chimbiri 2007; Dimbuene et al. 2014).

These everyday practices are also part of the traditional culture: in particular, when a man asks a woman or girl to have sex, the man must offer her resources in exchange. Wealthy men drive the sexual exchange, and have significantly higher levels of HIV, yet there are few, if any, NGO programmes that target men for behaviour change.

In my conversations with Malawians, the practice of *fisi* is invariably introduced. Yet as well as the absence of the epidemiological evidence to show that the *fisi* practice is of low risk, there is also a lack of evidence to suggest the *fisi* practice is widespread to the extent that it would significantly increase HIV prevalence rates in Malawi. When those in the NGO community who are concerned with *fisi* talk about it, they invariably refer to two of the 28 districts, Nsanje and Mangochi as examples. For example, a *fisi* (a male adult who has sexual intercourse with newly initiated girls) is uniquely practiced in societies such as among the Chewa and among the Yao in which their form of initiation for girls (called *chinamwali* and *chindakula* respectively) encourages sexual intercourse for initiates (Malawi Human Rights Commission 2006, p. 8). But we see also the role of *fisi* in widow cleansing, *fisi* for Procreation, Birth Cleansing (*kulimbitsa mwana*), Death Cleansing and for Cleansing Infidelity (Malawi Human Rights Commission 2006, p. 8). In my conversations with Malawians it was also assumed by them that the fisi was infected.

Although the *fisii* are involved in a variety of rituals, the NGOs focus on young girls, probably because so many of them are engaged in helping women and girls. I did not hear much about *fisi* and sexual cleansing for someone who died. It is also important to mention that the *fisii* are paid.

Further, there is a lack of anthropological evidence to argue that this practice contributes significantly to high HIV rates. Studies in Malawi (see, e.g., Skinner et al. 2013; Munthali et al. 2006; Munthali and Zulu 2007; Kamlongera 2007; Banda and Kunkeyani 2015) and several donor and government-funded studies on sexual cultural practices and AIDS in Malawi (Kornfield and Namate 1997; Matinga and McConville 2003; Malawi Human Rights Commission 2006; Kalipeni and Garrard 2004; College of Medicine 2005; Kadzandira and Zisiyana 2006; Chimombo 2006; Conroy et al. 2006) have been used to explain how sexual cultural practices are spreading HIV in Malawi, yet these results have been amplified outside these studies' findings.

Why is there then so much focus on something that in numerical terms at best has a minor effect on the increase of AIDS at a national level? The *fisi* practice does not contribute significantly to the spread of HIV for four reasons. First, epidemiological evidence reveals that the probability of infection during one heterosexual act is startlingly low.[3] Second, there is a lack of evidence to demonstrate how prevalent the practice is in Malawi. Third, although studies have been carried out on sexual cultural practices in Malawi, there is little empirical evidence to demonstrate that the *fisi* practice is contributing to the spread of HIV at a national scale. Fourth, although the emphasis on *fisi* in HIV discourse has been on poor young women (15–24) as drivers of the epidemic, HIV prevalence rates are higher in urban areas among women aged 30–34 who are in the highest wealth quintile in Malawi (Mishra et al. 2007). This category of women is significantly different from girls and young women living in rural areas aged 15 and below who may be participating in the *fisi* practice. This category of women is also different from widows where the term fisi is used for widow cleansing rites.

Narratives linking sexual cultural practices and HIV have been constructed which blame the *fisi* practice for the spread of AIDS. The *fisi* practice is being used as a scapegoat for three main reasons. First, the elites working in NGOs need constant donor funding. Thus, maintaining the *fisi* narrative to attract donor funding contributes to the stability of the policies and programmes directed to reduce transmission and thereby ensuring their jobs remain intact. Second, to project the issue of AIDS as a disease being spread by rural people, which detracts attention from the educated elite's sexual behaviour. Third, it supports a Christian narrative that sees those practising African Traditional Religion as backwards. This narrative has been amplified because it reflects the modernising agenda of key elites in Malawi, as opposed to reflecting a proportionate threat to the spread of AIDS. This deflects attention from high-risk sexual practices such as multiple sexual partners particularly among urban and affluent Malawians. AIDS policies should be designed to address contemporary patriarchal constructions of gender and power than a one-off highly un-evidenced traditional sexual practice. What I argue is there is evidence of a lack of evidence to support the policy to eradicate the practice of *fisi* because of the link with HIV.

THE ARGUMENT

In this book, I argue that a complex interplay of interests has led to the construction of the narrative that the sexual cultural practice of *fisi* contributes significantly to the spread of AIDS. I argue this complexity can be best understood through three sets of arguments.

The first and main argument is that a narrative of blame is maintained by national elites in Malawi, to ensure that HIV is kept on the development policy agenda within the institutions in which they work, thus attracting donor funding and retaining the elites' professional status and salaries. Although the elites are concerned about getting the virus, this blame narrative ensures that the target group for intervention is rural communities rather than the elites themselves. This argument complements the theoretical work of Mosse (2011) who has pioneered the use of what he terms *the ethnography of aid*, using this methodology to unravel the complex layers and actors that combine in the production of development policy and practice. Mosse (2011) highlights the importance of actor relationships in constructing policy, as well as emphasising the importance of policy in mediating social and professional relationships (2011, p. 10). Mosse builds on the work of Harper (1998) and Wood (1998) and describes actor relationships as 'complex relationships including negotiations over status, access, disciplinary points of view, team leadership struggles, conflict management or compliance with client frameworks defining what counts as knowledge' (2011, p. 10). In terms of policy, Mosse argues that 'policy ideas gain currency because they are socially appropriate....they can submerge ideological differences, allowing compromise, room for manoeuvre or multiple criteria of success, thus winning supporters by mediating different understandings of development' (2011, p. 11). Like Mosse, my study emphasises policy construction as a process mediated by those involved in the policy process as well as highlighting the importance of the policy itself. In my research, those mediating the process were the people I interviewed working on HIV prevention. The policy that these actors are mediating is that traditional sexual cultural practices should be eradicated because they argue these practices are the main driver of the HIV pandemic in Malawi. Additionally, Mosse asserts that:

> The interests of national elites and the electoral concerns of those in power affect the state's policy choices, sector priorities, and programs, with important consequences for the poor. Equally, well-intentioned sector reform programs can run aground where they challenge vested interests, and democratic reforms often have limited or unpredictable effect on power relations. (Mosse 2004, p. 51)

This is relevant as I argue that one reason national elites are able to influence the HIV policy agenda is related to the desire of donors—and the NGOs that they support-to be given a simple and rational explanation for high transmission that they can easily focus implementation around. Mosse (2011) also makes reference to international professionals who have to secure their positions within institutional and social contexts, which he says are hugely complex. Although Mosse in this context mainly refers to international professionals, I show that the same is true for national professionals working in development in Malawi, which means that groups of specialists and professionals need to sustain certain agendas to maintain their own status and positions. This argument is also linked to the work of Gibson et al. (2005) who argue that the structure of foreign aid can produce perverse outcomes that impede effectiveness and that the aid system is based on a set of power relations between actors ultimately driven by money.

These points are relevant to my argument: as I show in chapter four that organisations and agencies working on AIDS are major employers in Malawi. Although these development organisations are unlikely to disappear, they are also unstable as they rely on external funding. Successive themes come and go (e.g. HIV/AIDS, governance, gender, climate change) and with them jobs appear and disappear. Maintaining the narrative that the sexual cultural practice of *fisi* is spreading HIV can ensure policy and programmes directed to reduce HIV transmission continue. Today we see that interest in AIDS is declining so those working in NGOs are anxious: what would be the next 'big issue' that would support them?[4] This would most certainly be the case in many countries in sub-Saharan Africa that heavily depend on donors.

My second argument is that AIDS is presented by national, educated elites as a disease being spread by those living in rural areas, most of whom have little education beyond the first years of primary school and are often referred to by the elites as 'ignorant'. The narrative of sexual cultural practices thus absolves the educated elite from contributing to the epidemic as well as detracting attention from higher HIV prevalence rates in urban areas. This argument is situated within and supported by the literature on what is called 'the underdeveloped other' (Gramsci and Hoare 1971; Escobar 1988; Hobart 1993; Quarles van Ufford and Saleminck 2006). As I highlight in this book, this 'othering' is a result of those elites working in HIV prevention providing explanations to 'problems' that satisfy donors and therefore ensure continued funding. As a result, the educated elites who are perceived as civilised, distance themselves from rural people who they perceive as uncivilised. As Escobar (1995) asserts 'rather than being eliminated by development, many "traditional cultures" survive through their transformative engagement with modernity' (1995, p. 219). Elites in Malawi maintain their positions through their engagement with western discourses on modernity and distance themselves from Malawians living in rural areas who they perceive as backwards. The Malawian elites are making themselves look like the modern, unproblematic group that donors should work with.

The third argument is that the Malawian elites see those practising African Traditional Religion as backwards. Those who have converted to Christianity perceive themselves as modern and progressive. This argument has been guided by postcolonial theorists including Bassey (1999), Kitching (1982), Ngũgĩ wa Thiong'o (1986), and Lloyd (1967). They describe the elite in sub-Saharan Africa as the postcolonial elite as they have converted to Christianity. Postcolonial theory is thus relevant to my study as it follows on from the imperialist idea of westernising the backward. What it demonstrates is that the elites in Malawi are perpetuating an imperialist narrative by blaming people who practise African Traditional Religion as backwards, thereby establishing their modernity. Further,

Christianity allows them to be seen as consistent with western discourses on modernity.

I have presented three sets of arguments to explain why this narrative of blame is prevalent in Malawi, and these are interlocking. Several theories have influenced my argument: anthropology of development theory, postcolonial theory, theories on the policy process, elite theory and epidemiology. I will explore these theories in Chapter 2.

Malawi has suffered from one of the highest HIV prevalence rates in sub-Saharan Africa, with HIV prevalence among sexually active adults 15–49 years of age estimated at 10% (Joint United Nations Programme on HIV/AIDS [UNAIDS] 2013). It is also one of the poorest countries: its ranking on the UN's Human Development Index is 0.385, below the mean for sub-Saharan Africa of 0.389; and its per capita GNI is estimated at $911, below the mean for sub-Saharan Africa of $2050 (UN 2010). The population is predominantly rural (about 85%), and contains many ethnic groups with varying traditional cultural practices (Kornfield and Namate 1997; Matinga and McConville 2003; Malawi Human Rights Commission 2006). Particularly relevant for this research is the role of donors (Crewe and Harrison 1998; Mosse 2005). International donors (i.e. bi- and multilateral agencies) have been quite generous to Malawi (OECD-DAC 2007; UN 2006), perhaps in part due to its extreme poverty and the severity of its AIDS epidemic, as well as other health issues. Given its political stability, and the widespread use of English in government and the NGOs, Malawi is a relatively pleasant place for international aid workers to work which in part accounts for the large expatriate aid community.

At the time of my research, HIV prevalence rates in Malawi were higher in the south (20–22%) than the north (8%) and centre (7%); and higher in urban than rural areas (MDHS 2004). For example, while 18% of urban women are HIV positive, the corresponding proportion for rural women is 13%. For men, the urban–rural difference in HIV prevalence is even greater; men living in urban areas are nearly twice as likely to be infected than those living in rural areas (16 and 9%, respectively) (MDHS 2004, p. 231). As noted previously, this is very significant since sexual cultural practices are reported to be largely rural practices, yet HIV prevalence is lower in rural areas.

Further, although donors and NGOs have featured young women and girls between age 15 and 24 as particularly vulnerable to HIV in sub-Saharan Africa (UNAIDS 2004, p. 2), at the time of this study HIV prevalence in Malawi was higher among women aged 30–34 (18%) compared to 3.7% of women aged 15–19 (MDHS 2010). In addition, no data existed for HIV prevalence rates among girls under the age of 15. Women are tested at antenatal clinics, to which few girls under 15 would attend. And yet this is the demographic partaking in initiation ceremonies, which supports my argument that those blaming sexual cultural practices for the spread of HIV cannot support their case. In terms of education and wealth, HIV prevalence rates are highest among women with a secondary education and above (15.1%) compared to those women with no education (13.6%). In terms of income, those women with the highest rates of HIV were in the top wealth quintile.

Since the mid-1980s and the movement towards the privatisation of foreign aid, donor funding has been channeled to support NGOs. A study showed that the number of registered NGOs increased from a handful in 1964, at the time of Independence, to approximately 120 in 2003 (Morfit 2008). With the vast number of NGOs and development agencies operating in the country aid becomes tightly clustered resulting in and reinforcing the 'donor-darling'/'donor orphan' divide (Koch 2007). Registration of NGOs is incomplete, but a proxy measure—the sheer number of advertisements for NGO positions in the newspapers—shows a dramatic increase, as I anecdotally noted during my fieldwork in Malawi.

The NGO positions are filled by the Malawian elites. The international elites (with PhDs from abroad) and national elites (with university degrees) did not grow up in the rural areas and almost invariably did their schooling in Lilongwe or Blantyre (Watkins and Swidler 2013). The disparagement by the elites of harmful cultural practices is a way of establishing their modernity, ensuring distance from what they call the 'backward' rural areas. The NGO sector, although unlikely to disappear, is unstable, with successive themes coming and going (e.g. development, food security, gender)—and, with them, jobs appearing and disappearing. The elite seems aware of the way that their public statements on culture, on women's rights and on AIDS have pragmatic purposes in positioning them for new employment should their current jobs end. In other words, by maintaining a narrative of the blame for AIDS that focuses on harmful cultural practices the elite can ensure the stability of the policy and programmes directed to reduce transmission and their jobs remain intact.

THE CONTEXT

The main period of fieldwork for this study coincided with an exceptional moment in the Government of Malawi's response to AIDS. In 2006, the Law Commission received two submissions from the National AIDS Commission (NAC) and the Department of Nutrition, HIV/AIDS, requesting the development of legislative framework governing issues related to HIV/AIDS. A Special Law Commission was established in 2007, representing public and private sectors and people living with AIDS. A reform process started in 2007, when a decision was made to create new legislation rather than incorporate HIV/AIDS into existing pieces of legislation (P18).

Objectives of the legislation were to strengthen institutional structures dealing with HIV/AIDS; entrench human rights protection with respect to HIV/AIDS for those affected and infected; introduce criminal sanctions related to HIV infection or conduct and actions that promote infection; and consider entrenching the public health concerns relating to HIV/AIDS as a disease (Malawi Law Commission 2008). Broad areas covered by the legislation include the institutional framework; gender and HIV/AIDS; human rights and HIV/AIDS; education and HIV/AIDS; information and HIV/AIDS; public health and HIV/AIDS; employment and HIV/AIDS; and criminal law and HIV/AIDS (Malawi Law Commission 2008).

According to the Law Commission, 'the vulnerability of women and girls to HIV/AIDS is aggravated by certain cultural and religious practices' (2009, p. 33). The legislation intended to prohibit or regulate harmful practices that pose a risk of infection with HIV and other Sexually Transmitted Infections (STIs). It also addressed the issue of subjecting others to harmful practices. The Law Commission identified eighteen cultural practices. These include *Chiharo* (marrying the wife of a deceased brother); *Chimwanamaye* (exchanging of husbands or wives); *kulowa kufa* (cleansing after death). In my interviews, *respondents featured fisi*, which means 'hyena' in English, has two meanings. First, a man (who is referred to as *fisi*) is chosen by the village leader to have sex with young girls at initiation ceremonies. Second, a *fisi* can also be a man hired by a family to have sex with a married woman who cannot conceive, and therefore a secret arrangement is made with the *fisi* (see Chapter 4 for more details about the legislation).

These practices are considered to be contributing factors to the spread of AIDS (Kalipeni and Garrard 2004; College of Medicine 2005; Munthali et al. 2006; Kadzandira and Zisiyana 2006; Chimombo 2006; Conroy et al. 2006). The legislation referring to human rights proposes to prohibit discrimination on the basis of HIV/AIDS—whether perceived or actual—and to provide for rights of persons infected with HIV or suffering from AIDS. Finally, the criminal law legislation aims to create offences on deliberate transmission and to create differentiated categories from deliberate to negligent and reckless acts or omissions (Malawi Law Commission 2008).

Policies regarding sexual cultural practices became projects. Policies and projects are constructed by donors and by the Government of Malawi to eradicate or modify practices. They have vested interests and pursue their own agendas. Donors globally are pursuing the human rights agenda, promoting gender equality and the rights of women and girls, as set out by international frameworks such as the UN's Convention on the Elimination of all Forms of Discrimination Against Women. Donors think they are pursuing these policies in order to reduce AIDS in Malawi and thereby improving the health and well-being of the population: in particular that of girls and women subjected to these practices. The Government and NGOs' agenda is to maintain funding from donors so that the Malawian elites can hold on to their positions and the associated lifestyle.

Methodological Approach

The main aim of my research was to examine how policies on HIV prevention and harmful cultural practices have come to be linked. I identified five objectives to meet this aim. First, I assessed the extent to which the epistemic community in Malawi reframed the AIDS epidemic to further their goals and self-interests. Second, I investigated whether the debates within the epistemic community are facilitated or constrained by international donors (bi- and multilateral agencies). Third, I explored whether or not AIDS is being represented as an exceptional circumstance, justifying policies that would not normally be applied to other public health crises, for example, STIs such as gonorrhoea or syphilis. Fourth, I examined the extent to which international frameworks, agendas and paradigms are influencing and impacting on traditional cultural practices and women's rights, resulting in changes to legislation to ban such practices. And finally, I assessed the implications of the findings for the conceptualisation and provision of future and current AIDS policies and programmes in Malawi. The overall rationale for these research questions is that future HIV prevention programmes will be more effective and based on rigorous scientific evidence.

I identified five research questions to complete this study: (i) how are epistemic communities framing and/or reframing the AIDS epidemic to further their goals and self-interests (such as keeping themselves in jobs)?; (ii) how are the debates within the epistemic community facilitated or constrained by international donors (bi- and multilateral agencies)?; (iii) to what extent are HIV/AIDS being represented as exceptional circumstances, justifying policies that would not normally be applied to different public health crises?; (iv) how are international frameworks, agendas and paradigms influencing and impacting on traditional cultural practices and women's rights, resulting in changes to legislation to ban such practices?; and (v) what are the implications for AIDS policies and programmes in Malawi?

The data emerges from research in Malawi from 2008–2009. In order to understand how constructions of narratives linking AIDS and sexual cultural practices came about, I conducted 60 in-depth interviews in four districts: Balaka ($n = 15$), Blantyre ($n = 7$), Lilongwe ($n = 34$), and Zomba ($n = 4$)—with expatriates and Malawians working on HIV prevention including lawyers, researchers, policymakers, government ministers, NGO staff, national and district officials and health workers. I interviewed 39 men and 21 women. All respondents were Chewa.

I asked questions relating to themselves, their profession and what they liked and disliked about it, to find out about their lives as development professionals. Questions then focused on the themes of cultural practices, gender and AIDS to find out to what extent they thought cultural practices contributed to the spread of AIDS. I used snowball sampling to identify respondents which enabled them to be easily identifiable, willing to be interviewed and generous with suggestions of others to interview. Having positioned myself in one of the biggest AIDS NGOs in Malawi for several months, it was relatively straightforward to identify respondents at an early stage.

Interviews were either recorded or I made notes and transcribed. Analysis of interview transcripts and field notes took an inductive approach and data were analysed adopting elements from grounded theory. These 60 in-depth interviews were the main data source used in this book and these data were coded; patterns in the data identified by means of thematic codes and each code compared to other codes to identify similarities and differences. I coded for key issues (*fisi*, what respondent say are bad about cultural practices, what they say in a general way about harmful cultural practices, their religion and ethnicity). Key issues emerged as a result of reading the interview transcripts many times and these issues became the major findings of the wider study.

These data were one component of a wider ethnography. I lived with Malawian development professionals, kept journal notes, visited two main newspaper headquarters and photocopied newspaper articles spanning 10 years covering stories on AIDS. Further I collected policy documents (which were often difficult to get hold of), attended meetings and conferences in Malawi and talked to many people. I worked as a consultant for UNAIDS to see how organisations' AIDS policies were 'harmonised and aligned' with Malawi's HIV prevention strategy, for which I conducted 28 semi-structured interviews with people working on HIV prevention. These data fed into my overall findings. The argument I present in this book is evidenced by my critical analysis of interviews, newspaper articles, policy documents as well as secondary academic sources.

I aligned my research with the interpretivist paradigm to include ontological, epistemological and methodological assumptions as acknowledged by Guba and Lincoln (1994, pp. 107–108). According to Mertens, 'a researcher's theoretical orientation has implications for every decision made in the research process, including the choice of method' (2005, pp. 3–4). Methods traditionally associated with the interpretivist approach are mainly qualitative and can include participant observation, focus group discussions, action research, ethnography, phenomenology and discourse analysis. A qualitative rather than a quantitative approach was therefore undertaken for this research as I investigate the opinions, interpretations, beliefs, values and attitudes of agencies rather than the collection of statistical data. This approach also enabled the collection of rich data to critique the response to HIV prevention in Malawi at the time the fieldwork took place.

Qualitative research methods were the main methods used in this study. I decided to use qualitative methods because I conducted research on people's views on AIDS and sexual cultural practices, therefore it was necessary to look at the social, political and cultural factors which may influence a person's view. The best way to obtain data to analyse the impact of such factors is the use of methods such as participant observation or ethnographic research. This approach allows the researcher to get inside the skin of his or her research subjects. The researcher is then taking on more of a learning role as opposed to a scientific testing role (Silverman 1993) as s/he is observing the situation in context. This approach also allowed me to obtain data that cannot be retrieved by using methods typically associated with positivism (e.g. statistical modelling or fixed choice questions to random samples).

STRUCTURE OF THE BOOK

I start with a review of how others have thought and written about elites and policymaking. Those readers interested only in the findings of the study on which this book is based could skip straight to Chapter 3 (though they would miss out on some theoretical insights which help to make meaning of the results which follow).

In Chapter 2 I present theoretical perspectives that have informed the study. Due to the interdisciplinary nature of this research, I show how a number of theories influenced by argument. First, using the approaches used within the anthropology of development I provide a critique of HIV policymaking. Second, and in order to understand how policy was constructed based on misconceptions, I draw on elite and policymaking theories to demonstrate how the policy process is being mediated by the agendas of elites as opposed to bio-medical facts. Third, I use postcolonial theory to highlight how the elites are interpreting for themselves the colonial narrative that is founded on a binary opposition; civilised (the elites) and the uncivilised (the rural uneducated population). This then enables the elites to distance themselves from those living in rural areas, allowing them to maintain a position of power and access to the resources flowing in from the aid community.

In Chapter 3 *The Development Aid Situation in Malawi*, I provide a brief history of the development aid situation, which is given to highlight the reliance of the National Government on external aid to address high prevalence rates. I then demonstrate how the HIV pandemic is widely considered an emergency and I highlight how AIDS has been represented as an exceptional circumstance, justifying policies that are unique to this country's context. I analyse HIV and harmful cultural practices in Malawi and explain how, given the epidemiology of HIV, the *fisi* practice cannot account for the spread of the epidemic.

In Chapter 4 *Harmful Cultural Practices' and AIDS*, I show how what are called 'harmful cultural practices' have emerged as a development issue in global conventions and policies over the past ten years. I then analyse the shift from the global to the national level and demonstrate how international policy has influenced national policy on harmful cultural practices and AIDS in Malawi. I use data to show how the Malawian elite have constructed narratives of blame concerning AIDS and cultural practices which reflect their view that the backwardness of village people is to blame for high HIV prevalence rates.

In Chapter 5 *How the Church Frames AIDS*, I explore the link between religion and AIDS and analyse the influence of the church in shaping the views of the Malawian elite. I demonstrate through my interviews how the attendance of Malawian elites at church has influenced the way they think about AIDS, cultural practices and rural people. First, I provide the religious context in Malawi. I explore how religious elites perceive cultural practices as negative and backward, positioned against their Christian beliefs they perceive as enlightened.

In Chapter 6 *The Construction of Policy: Donors, AIDS and Sexual Cultural Practices*, I analyse the policy construction process and review literature on policymaking processes, concluding that the policymaking process is messy and complex. I argue that stakeholders try to influence HIV policy by using narratives and discourses to pursue their own vested interests, which are presented as knowledge. Additionally, I look at the aid game in Malawi. I then consider how these narratives have been passed on through education. I review donors' perceptions of harmful cultural practices and argue that donors have absorbed narratives of blame linking harmful cultural practices and AIDS because it feeds into and supports the dominant neocolonialist view of the African other as primitive and backward.

In Chapter 7 *Conclusion and Recommendations*, I argue that my ethnographic approach has enabled me to highlight how 'narratives of blame' are used as a smokescreen to pursue government and donors' interests. I also present policy recommendations and suggestions for future research.

NOTES

1. For example researchers at MLSFH presented the NAC with their findings on AIDS. They probably never read them as they have to follow donors, not researchers.
2. For example, Ghana; Amoakohene (2004). Kenya; Oluga et al. (2010) and Ayikukwei et al. (2008). Mali; Mackie and LeJeune (2009). Mozambique; Kotanyi and Krings-Ney (2009). Nigeria; Adesina (2015). Sierra Leone; M'jamtu-Sie (2007). South Africa; Oluga et al. (2010). South Africa, Lesotho, and Swaziland; (UNICEF 2003). Tanzania; Wadesango et al. (2011) and Oluga et al. (2010). Uganda; Asiimwe et al. (2003). Zambia; Moyo and Müller (2011).
3. Early in the epidemic Gray et al. (2001) estimated probability of infection at 0.001. Thus, out of a 1000 people who are not infected with HIV, for every act of unprotected intercourse with a person one is HIV positive.
4. See Norma Anderson (2017) who argues that when development trends and issues in Malawi change, at donors' wishes, organisations proactively strategize to vie for donors. Her data show that between 2008 and 2010 there was a widespread belief among civil society in Malawi that climate change was becoming the 'it' issue, surpassing HIV/AIDS in predominance.

REFERENCES

Adesina, M. O. (2015). Trado-cultural practices, situation, analysis and epidemiological factors in the spread of HIV/AIDS in Nigeria. *Journal of Education and Practice*, 6(21), 65–70.

Amoakohene, M. I. (2004). Violence against women in Ghana: A look at women's perceptions and review of policy and social responses. *Social Science and Medicine*, 59(11), 2373–2385.

Anderson, N. J. (2017). Ephemeral development agendas and the process of priority shifts in Malawi. *Journal of Asian and African Studies*, 52(7), 915–931.

Asiimwe, D., Kibombo, R., & Neema, S. (2003). *Focus group discussions on social cultural factors impacting on HIV/AIDS in Uganda*. Kampala: Makerere Institute of Social Research.

Ayikukwei, R., Ngare, D., Sidle, J., Ayuku, D., Baliddawa, J., & Greene, J. (2008). HIV/AIDS and cultural practices in western Kenya: The impact of sexual cleansing rituals on sexual behaviours. *Culture, Health & Sexuality*, 10(6), 587–599.

Banda, F., & Kunkeyani, T. E. (2015). Renegotiating cultural practices as a result of HIV in the eastern region of Malawi. *Culture, Health & Sexuality*, 17(1), 34–47.

Bassey, M. O. (1999). *Western education and political domination in Africa: A study in critical and dialogical pedagogy*. Westport, CT: Bergin and Garvey.

Boily, M.-C., Baggaley, R. F., Wang, L., Masse, B., White, R. G., Hayes, R. J., et al. (2009). Heterosexual risk of HIV-1 infection per sexual act: Systematic review and meta-analysis of observational studies. *The Lancet Infectious Diseases, 9*(2), 118–129.

Chimbiri, A. (2007). The condom is an 'intruder' in marriage: Evidence from rural Malawi. *Social Science & Medicine, 64*(5), 1102–1115.

Chimombo, S. (2006). *The hyena wears darkness*. Zomba: WASI Publications.

Chizimba, R., et al. (2004). The development and implementation of the national behaviour change interventions strategy for HIV/AIDS/SRH in Malawi: An evidence-based approach to planning strategic behaviour change interventions. National AIDS Commission, Malawi.

College of Medicine. (2005). *Cultural practices related to sexual and reproductive health outcomes and HIV transmission*. Blantyre: College of Medicine.

Conroy, A., Blackie, M., Whiteside, A., Malewezi, J., & Sachs, J. (2006). *Poverty, AIDS and hunger: Breaking the poverty trap in Malawi*. Hampshire: Palgrave Macmillan.

Coombes, Y. (2001). *A literature review to support the situational analysis for the national behaviour change interventions strategy on HIV/AIDS and sexual and reproductive health*. London: DFID.

Crewe, E., & Harrison, E. (1998). *Whose development? An ethnography of aid*. London: Zed.

Dimbuene, Z. T., Emina, J. B., & Sankoh, O. (2014). UNAIDS 'multiple sexual partners' core indicator: Promoting sexual networks to reduce potential biases. *Global Health Action, 7*(1), 23103.

Escobar, A. (1988). Power and visibility: Development and the intervention and management of the third world. *Cultural Anthropology, 3*(4), 428–443.

Escobar, A. (1995). *Encountering development: The making and unmaking of the third world*. Princeton, NJ: Princeton University Press.

Gibson, C. C., Andersson, K., Ostrom, E., & Shivakumar, S. (2005). *The Samaritan's dilemma: The political economy of development aid*. Oxford: Oxford University Press on Demand.

Gramsci, A., & Hoare, Q. (1971). *Selections from the prison notebooks* (Vol. 294). London: Lawrence and Wishart.

Gray, R. H., Wawer, M. J., Brookmeyer, R., Sewankambo, N. K., Serwadda, D., Wabwire-Mangen, F., ... & Quinn, T. C. (2001). Probability of HIV-1 transmission per coital act in monogamous, heterosexual, HIV-1-discordant couples in Rakai, Uganda. *The Lancet, 357*(9263), 1149–1153.

Guba, E. G., & Lincoln, Y. S. (1994). Competing paradigms in qualitative research. *Handbook of Qualitative Research, 2*(163–194), 105.

Haas, P. M. (1992). Epistemic communities and international policy coordination: Introduction. *International Organisation, 46*(1), 1–35.

Harper, R. H. (1998). *Inside the IMF: An ethnography of documents, technology and organisational action*. London and New York: Routledge.

Hobart, M. (1993). *An anthropological critique of development: The growth of ignorance*. London: Routledge.

Joint United Nations Programme on HIV/AIDS (UNAIDS). (2013). *Progress report on the global plan towards the elimination of new HIV infections among children by 2015 and keeping their mothers alive*. Geneva: UNAIDS.

Kadzandira, J. M., & Zisiyana, C. (2006). *Assessment of risk practices and sites where such practices take place in the urban areas of Lilongwe and Blantyre districts*. Zomba: Centre for Social Research.

Kalipeni, E., & Garrard, C. (Eds.). (2004). *HIV/AIDS in Africa: Beyond epidemiology*. Oxford and Cambridge: Blackwell.

Kamlongera, A. (2007). What becomes of 'her'? A look at the Malawian fisi culture and its effects on young girls. *Agenda, 21*(74), 81–87.

Kitching, G. (1982). *Development and underdevelopment in historical perspective*. New York: Methuen.

Koch, D. J. (2007). Uncharted territories: The geographical choices of aid agencies. *The Broker, 1*(3), 9–12.

Kornfield, R. & Namate, D. (1997). *Cultural practices related to HIV/AIDS risk behaviour: Community survey in Phalombe, Malawi* (No. 10). Support to AIDS and Family Health (STAFH) Project 612-238.

Kotanyi, S., & Krings-Ney, B. (2009). Introduction of culturally sensitive HIV prevention in the context of female initiation rites: An applied anthropological approach in Mozambique. *African Journal of AIDS Research, 8*(4), 491–502.

Lloyd, P. C. (1967). *Africa in social change: Changing traditional societies in the modern world*. Baltimore: Penguin Books.

Mackie, G., & LeJeune, J. (2009). *Social dynamics of abandonment of harmful practices: A new look at the theory* (Innocenti Working Paper No. XXX). Florence: UNICEF Innocenti Research Centre.

Malawi Demographic and Health Survey. (2004). Maryland: NSO and ORC Macro.

Malawi Human Rights Commission. (2006). *Cultural practices and their impact on the enjoyment of human rights, particularly the rights of women and children in Malawi*. MHRC: Malawi.

Malawi Law Commission. (2008). *Report of the Law Commission on the development of HIV and AID legislation*. Lilongwe: Malawi.

Matinga, P., & McConville, F. (2003). *A review of cultural beliefs and practices influencing sexual and reproductive health and health-seeking behaviour, in Malawi*. Malawi: Department for International Development (DFID).

Mertens, D. M. (2005). *Research methods in education and psychology: Integrating diversity with quantitative and qualitative approaches* (2nd ed.). Thousand Oaks: Sage.

Mishra, V., Bignami-Van Assche, S., Greener, R., Vaessen, M., Hong, R., Ghys, P. D., et al. (2007). HIV infection does not disproportionately affect the poorer in sub-Saharan Africa. *AIDS, 21*(Supp.7), S17–S28.

M'jamtu-Sie, N. (2007). The impact of culture and tradition on attitudes to health in Sierra Leone. *Journal of Hospital Librarianship, 6*(4), 93–107.

Morfit, S. (2008). *Dangerous development: The global response to AIDS in Africa*. Unpublished Master's Paper, Department of Sociology, University of California, Berkeley.

Morfit, N. S. (2011). "AIDS is money": How donor preferences reconfigure local realities. *World Development, 39*(1), 64–76.

Mosse, D. (2004). Is good policy unimplementable? Reflections on the ethnography of aid policy and practice. *Development and Change, 35*(4), 639–671.

Mosse, D. (2005). *Cultivating development: An ethnography of aid policy and practice*. London & Ann Arbor, MI: Pluto Press.

Mosse, D. (2011). Introduction: The anthropology of expertise and professionals in international development. In D. Mosse (Ed.), *Adventures in Aidland*. Oxford: Berghahn Books.

Moyo, N., & Müller, J. C. (2011). The influence of cultural practices on the HIV and AIDS pandemic in Zambia. *HTS Theological Studies, 67*(3), 412–417.

Munthali, A. C., & Zulu, E. M. (2007). The timing and role of initiation rites in preparing young people for adolescence and responsible sexual and reproductive behaviour in Malawi. *African Journal of Reproductive Health, 11*(3), 150.

Munthali A. C., Moore, A., Konyani, S., & Zakeyo, B. (2006). *Qualitative evidence of adolescents' sexual and reproductive health experiences in selected districts of Malawi*. New York: The Alan Guttmacher Guttmacher Institute.

Myroniuk, T. W. (2011). Global discourses and experiential speculation: Secondary and tertiary graduate Malawians dissect the HIV/AIDS epidemic. *Journal of the International AIDS Society, 14*(1), 47.

NSO, M., & Macro, I. C. F. (2011). *Malawi demographic and health survey 2010*. Zomba, Malawi and Calverton, MD: NSO and ORC Macro.

OECD-DAC, D. A. C. (2007). *Action-Oriented Policy Paper on Human Rights and Development*.

Oluga, M., Kiragu, S., Mohamed, M. K., & Walli, S. (2010). 'Deceptive' cultural practices that sabotage HIV/AIDS education in Tanzania and Kenya. *Journal of Moral Education, 39*(3), 365–380.

Quarles van Ufford, P., & Saleminck, O. (2006). *After the fall: Cosmopolitanism and the paradoxical politics of global inclusion and authenticity*. Paper prepared for the panel on cosmopolitanism and development. Association of Social Anthropologists Diamond Jubilee Conference, Keele, UK.

Silverman, D. (1993). *Interpreting qualitative data*. London: Sage.

Skinner, J., Underwood, C., Schwandt, H., & Magombo, A. (2013). Transitions to adulthood: Examining the influence of initiation rites on the HIV risk of adolescent girls in Mangochi and Thyolo districts of Malawi. *AIDS Care, 25*(3), 296–301.

Smith, K. P., & Watkins, S. C. (2005). Perceptions of risk and strategies for prevention: Responses to HIV/AIDS in rural Malawi. *Social Science and Medicine, 60*(3), 649–660.

UN. (2006). *Human Development Report.* New York: UN.

UN. (2010). *Human Development Report.* New York: UN.

UNAIDS. (2004). *Women and HIV/AIDS: Confronting the crisis.* Geneva: UNAIDS.

UNICEF. (2003). *Child protection: An analysis and achievements in 2003.* New York: UNICEF.

Wa Thiong'o, N. (1986). *Decolonizing the mind: The politics of language in African literature.* London: Heinemann Educational Books.

Wadesango, N., Rembe, S., & Chabaya, O. (2011). Violation of women's rights by harmful traditional practices. *The Anthropologist, 13*(2), 121–129.

Watkins, S. C., & Swidler, A. (2009). Hearsay ethnography: Conversational journals as a method for studying culture in action. *Poetics, 37*(2), 162–184.

Watkins, S. C., & Swidler, A. (2013). Working misunderstandings: Donors, brokers, and villagers in Africa's AIDS industry. *Population and Development Review, 38,* 197–218.

Wood, P. (1998). *The rise of consultancy and the prospect for regions.* Paper presented at the 38th congress of the European Regional Science Association, Vienna, 28–31.

Open Access This chapter is licensed under the terms of the Creative Commons Attribution 4.0 International License (http://creativecommons.org/licenses/by/4.0/), which permits use, sharing, adaptation, distribution and reproduction in any medium or format, as long as you give appropriate credit to the original author(s) and the source, provide a link to the Creative Commons licence and indicate if changes were made.

The images or other third party material in this chapter are included in the chapter's Creative Commons licence, unless indicated otherwise in a credit line to the material. If material is not included in the chapter's Creative Commons licence and your intended use is not permitted by statutory regulation or exceeds the permitted use, you will need to obtain permission directly from the copyright holder.

CHAPTER 2

Theoretical Perspectives

This chapter provides an overview of the literature relevant to my three sets of arguments. My theoretical framework has been influenced by scholars within anthropology of development as I provide a critique of a specific policy field in development. It exposes current misconceptions among development practitioners and policymakers in Malawi concerning AIDS: that sexual cultural practices are fuelling the HIV pandemic. I argue that this is an example of a development policy and programme that has failed. Thus, literature within the field of anthropology of development, especially the work of Mosse (2011) and Crewe and Harrison (1998) is relevant because their research demonstrates how many different actors are involved in influencing policies and programmes. They critically analyse the complex relationships of power between global multilateral organisations, donors, governments of resource-poor countries, and local communities, and their impact on development projects. I also criticise the impact multilateral agencies have on development. I criticise the neoliberal economic ideology that has been used by agencies such as the World Bank and the International Monetary Fund (IMF) to offer financial assistance to low income countries. I critique this model of development and agree with Sadasivam (1997) and Macleans, Geo-Jaja and Mangum (2001) who argue that neoliberalism required low income countries to reduce spending on social issues including health, education and development, while debt repayment and other economic policies were prioritised. I also agree with Stiglitz (2000) who argues that

© The Author(s) 2019
S. Page, *Development, Sexual Cultural Practices and HIV/AIDS in Africa*, https://doi.org/10.1007/978-3-030-04119-9_2

25

institutions such as the IMF undermine democratic processes by imposing policies on national governments.

Mosse and Crewe also demonstrate how to critically engage with development practice by combining academic development work with academic writing and reflection, which is the praxis through which my research was produced. I have done this by working as a development practitioner while conducting my doctorate research. I worked as a consultant for UNAIDS in Malawi while doing my field work. Their approaches have been instrumental in helping me develop my own theoretical framework, as my research looks at how different people working within the field of AIDS are able to construct policies based on their own agendas while at the same time I questioned my own position as a researcher.

One area that is also particularly significant is that public policy making, particularly in terms of HIV prevention, is being set by the agendas of a group of elites (see section on elites in Chapter 6). Elite theory has its roots in the work of Pareto (1935) and Mosca (1896, 1939). They argued that society is governed and controlled by the interests of a group of powerful elites as opposed to the electorate. Such theorists reject an idealised notion of democracy as a reflection of the will of the people, instead arguing that a group of powerful elites own the decision-making power in government, corporations, and institutions that shape policy, and in doing so they act in accordance to their own self-interest. Pareto argued that there is a group of elites who control wealth and power until they are removed by a new aristocratic class (1935).

C. Wright Mills used elite theory to understand the nature of power in 1950s America. Mills (1956) argues that the structure of American society was such that a small hierarchy of groups monopolised power (Mills 1956) and that power is concentrated in several fields of life, including family, religion, education, professional life, military and politics (Mills 1956, p. 3). Mills uses the idea of the power elites in an attempt to overcome the over determinism of Marxism. For Mills, there is a range of elites who may have competing and conflicting interests, as opposed to power being centralised by a single group. This was the case with Marxist ideology where power was controlled by a single group 'the Bourgeoisie' and based on the ownership of the means of production (Marx and Engels 1962 first published 1848). Whereas Mills argues power is not held simply by one group, he also rejects pluralistic theory stating that the majority of these elites are interlocking and self-perpetuating (Mills 1956). Many individuals in such elite circles are democratically elected. Mills adds that they are not always conscious they are part of the elite. Lasswell and Kaplan (1950) in *Power and Society* remark that elites can hold more than one powerful position.

> Persons who occupy a top position with respect to one value are likely to hold correspondingly favourable positions with respect to other values; in fact, this possibility is the agglutination hypothesis. (Lasswell and Kaplan 1950, p. 97).

This theory has since been used in sociopolitical theory to describe any small group of people that controls a disproportionate amount of wealth, privileges, and access to decision-making (Bottomore 1993). Higley and Burton (2006) identify two elite types; united and disunited political elites and their associated political regimes. They define political elites as:

> persons who are able, by virtue of their authoritative positions in powerful organizations and movements of whatever kind, to affect national political outcomes regularly and substantially. (Higley and Burton 1989, p. 9).

Despite differences between elite theorists all conclude that power in society is monopolised by a small group of individuals or groups who shape or influence decisions that affect policy. The next section looks at how elites influence policy.

ELITE THEORY AND POLICYMAKING

Elite theory applied to policy making argues that policymaking is not simply based on using empirical research to construct the most effective means of dealing with a given social issue. Instead in reality any such policymaking process is mediated by a range of powerful elites, vying for their own interests, many of which may hold agendas that are quite contradictory to the objective aims of such policies. Anderson (1984) argues that the ruling elites create the narratives on which polices are constructed. Scholars such as Herrera (1996) concur with Anderson and argue that elites play a key role in defining problems and setting agendas for public policy making. In many contexts policies are shaped by elites who warp democratic processes. Lasswell (1936) argues political elites are able to do this through occupying key leadership positions, giving them proximity to power and resources, which they use to determine who gets what, when and how. He argues that as a result there is a clash between interests of the elite and those of the general public.

Easton (1965) in his major theoretical work *A Framework for Political Analysis* argued that most policy decisions concerning the allocation of scarce resources are made by the political elite in line with their interests. De Waal (1997) argues that the power of the elites working on humanitarian issues has been an obstacle to development. He refers to the 'internal political decay' in Africa, which along with increasing authoritarianism, has impeded the construction of anti-famine political contracts (1997, p. 3). He argues that NGOs tend to conflate their interests with those of 'the poor' and present their interests as identical. He reveals there are many organisational imperatives that drive NGO decisions and these are unrelated to the needs of the people whose lives they are trying to improve. In other words, their interests are not the same.

Mosse's (2011, p. 10) and Chin's (2007) work is also relevant. Mosse (2011) highlights the importance of actor relationships in the shaping and salience of policy ideas and the importance of policy ideas in maintaining professionals' jobs. In the context in which I worked policy ideas are both the policies and legislation drafted to eradicate sexual cultural practices in Malawi. However Mosse does not reduce policymaking processes to this alone. Chin (2007) concludes that AIDS policies and programmes are being implemented for social and moral reasons to keep the disease on the political agenda and, by implication, ensure funding and jobs for those working on HIV (Chin 2007 as cited by Whiteside and Smith 2009). Here it is important to note that the elites in Malawi have not manufactured a crisis, but instead they are shaping how this crisis is being interpreted to pursue their own agendas. In the context of Malawi, although policies on AIDS are not produced in national vacuums, they are informed by international frameworks and agendas: elites within Malawi have the power to warp such agendas for their own interests.

ELITES IN SUB-SAHARAN AFRICA

There is a wealth of literature on SSA that recognises that groups of elites play an important role in controlling power within national contexts (Svanikier 2007 and see Ornett and Hewitt 2006 for a comprehensive literature review on elites and institutions in SSA). SSA is diverse and it is perhaps unjust to make generalisations about the elites. However, Hossain and Moore provide a definition of the elites in a low income country context as:

> the people who make or shape the main political and economic decisions: ministers and legislators; owners and controllers of TV and radio stations and major business enterprises and activities; large property owners; upper-level public servants; senior members of the armed forces, police and intelligence services; editors of major newspapers; publicly prominent intellectuals, lawyers and doctors; and—more variably—influential socialites and heads of large trades unions, religious establishments and movements, universities and development NGOs ... In most developing countries, governing elites tend to be especially powerful. They often command a particularly large slice of the national income, and the influence that goes with it. (Hossain and Moore 2002, p. 1)

The many different national contexts in SSA imply that elites are not a homogenous group and indeed many scholars differentiate between the elites. Ornett and Hewitt (2006) remark that the elites are divided by ethnicity, functionality, politics and economics. They do not, however, divide the elites in terms of gender. They contend that since decolonisation, the elites in Africa have developed within or in close proximity to the state, as both politics and economics have been almost entirely linked to the state in countries in SSA.

In SSA it is important to highlight that the middle class is often absent as Sklar (1999) refers to the lack of an 'autonomous bourgeoisie' in most post-colonial African countries. However, In *Architects of Poverty*, Mbeki (2009) discusses the flawed capitalism in Africa and particularly censures the political elite, who he argues have no capital of their own and who manage to keep their fellow citizens poor while enriching themselves.

However Chandra (2006) argues that there is a middle class in Africa. She identifies elites as those who have the capital to launch a political career, who are upwardly mobile middle-class individuals, better educated and better off than the voters whom they seek to mobilise. She uses the term 'elite' interchangeably with the terms 'politician', 'candidate', 'incumbent' and 'entrepreneur' (Chandra 2006). Scholars such as Bassey (1999), Kitching (1982), Wa Thiong'o (1992), and Lloyd (1967) describe the elite in SSA as the postcolonial elite. They identify two types of postcolonial elites: elites with a Western style of education that enabled them to access employment opportunities with adequate wages to meet their living expenses; and elites associated with chiefs and administrative positions during the colonial period who had already acquired some wealth. They argue that in general both types of elites often shared some common Western behaviour patterns and had often converted to Christianity. The identification of Christianity as a factor in the identity of elites in SAA is particularly relevant in the findings of my study. Christianity not only plays a symbolic role in identifying commonality between high status individuals in Malawi but also was a driving force behind the policy construction of sexual cultural practices.

Galtung (1971) in his structural imperialism theory also focuses on the elite in terms of postcolonialism. He described the African elites as having more in common with Western elites than with 'their own people' thus sustaining neocolonialism in their quest for survival. In other words, the African elites are legitimising their existence within western contexts by converting to Christianity and by distancing themselves from the rest of their nation. Although some of these groups are not inherently political, divides between spheres of power, for example the business, the political, the religious in the Global South are far more porous.

Diop (2012) also refers to the self-interest of the new African modernising classes during the post-colonial period:

> The immediate post-colonial period was one of optimism in which the new African modernising classes had the opportunity to pick and choose the optimal modalities for development. But they failed to deliver, mesmerised as they were by the material dazzle of the products of modern market capitalism. But modern market capitalism needs and wants those products which in their raw forms serve as the basis for the production of those goods coveted by the post-colonial African bourgeoisie. The result of this class egotism is the open face of an Africa plagued by cultural collapse in key areas such as its vaunted communitarianism, only to be replaced by the false consciousness of corrosive self-interest, consumer greed, eruptive xenophobia – as in the cases of South Africa and Ivory Coast – and political corruption. (Diop 2012, p. 234).

Further he talks about elites in relation to their traditional cultures:

> The reader must have noticed that the word 'elites' is in the plural. In so doing I want to express the idea that all elites are concerned here:

intellectual, political, cultural, and those of the business world. The reason is that each particular elite group is necessarily imbued with the cultural tokens of tradition. But what creates the cultural antinomies is the fact that – for the most part – they willingly allow themselves to succumb to the temptations and blandishments of neoliberal capitalism. And in spite of the communitarian principles of their traditional cultures, the dictates of neoliberalism force them to satisfy their own individual wants and needs and not extend such privileges beyond their neo-class boundaries. (Diop 2012, p. 223)

Chabal and Daloz (1999) concur that that power is often exercised in SSA between Big men, or patrons, and their constituent communities (1999, p. 37). As a result, they hold the view that most state institutions in a number of countries have been subordinated to the interests of these elites. Several scholars also use the 'big man' model, a term made popular by Sahlins (1963), which in a SSA context describes the leader of a country who uses his networks to maintain power. The big man concept can be seen in Malawi and elsewhere in SSA as Cammack et al. (2006) points out there is a continuity in leadership style among Malawi's 'big men' and that the former President Mutharika was one of the big men (the President at the time the fieldwork for this study was conducted). Malawi has been considered a neopatrimonial state since its independence in 1964 and the 'big man syndrome' has been a perpetual feature of its politics. Cammack et al. (2007) conducted a study on the former President Mutharika and explains:

In 'hybrid' states where neopatrimonial politics are the norm there is by definition a weak legal regime. In such states the constitution, rules, laws, and behavioural norms may be well-articulated, even written down, but they are weakly applied. The institutions normally responsible for their application are themselves weak – judiciaries, watch-dog institutions, parliaments, police, media, civic organisations, etc. They are sometimes 'captured' by the leader through his control of the appointment (and dismissal) process, or through patronage and clientelist practices. States such as these are invariably poor and unproductive – because the weak regulatory environment makes them risky environments for investment and corrupt. Also, because they are unproductive, individuals are unlikely to have outside sources of income, or alternative economic prospects, and are therefore reliant on the leader (or one of his subordinates) for employment and income. When he uses the same techniques to get his way, there are few who can rein him in and no institutions to call upon to limit his excesses. (Cammack et al. 2007, p. 1)

Cammack et al. (2007) also makes an important point and remarks that the dynamics of neo-patrimonial politics tend to legitimise and strengthen elite groups that are not necessarily interested in focusing on development and subsequently accelerate the disparities even in states with sufficient capacity to fight poverty. Lange et al. (2000) focus on government elites in Tanzania setting up 'independent' civil society organisations (CSOs). They argue that these CSOs were staffed by civil servants to access funding from donors who, during the 1980s, turned to CSOs to take on the service delivery role that the state often failed to carry out as well as becoming more engaged in the policy process.

Although there is a vast literature on the elites in sub-Saharan Africa there are gaps in the body of knowledge concerning AIDS and the elites. One of the few scholars that addresses the subject is Van de Walle (2003). He argues that:

> The development of the pandemic defects the stability of the governing elite. All countries are run by a relatively small group of people who dominate government, party, army, business and civil society... One of the challenges facing many African countries is how to ensure a smooth transition from a relatively closed elite... to a more institutionalized and pluralistic system with wider access. The HIV/AIDS pandemic has several consequences. It erodes the institutionalization of the government and accelerates the need to replenish this elite. As noted, this affects patrimonial structures as well as rational-legal ones. Men and women who have decades of political experience, strong networks and respected judgment, are being lost, and younger cadres are being promoted to fill the posts, but cannot fill the structural gap... the most probable scenario is that those in power rely more heavily on a smaller circle of loyal comrades, and use more ruthless or corrupt methods to co-opt or buy support. (Van de Walle 2003, p. 300)

I also argue that there are a small group of elites in Malawi who dominate government and civil society in the context of policy making on AIDS.

Orrnert and Hewitt (2006) state that in small countries in Sub-Saharan Africa like in Malawi or Benin the number of elites can be very small (between 800 and 1000). And in larger countries like South Africa and Nigeria they will have more but in all cases the number of elites comprises a small portion of the population. Swidler and Watkins (2009) conducted research on the elites in Malawi and identified three types;

local elites, interstitial elites and national elites. Matiki (2001) remarks that the English language is used in Malawi to provide a code, which symbolises modernisation and elitism. Miller (1974) also makes the link between education and elitism and describes education as being the pathway to elite status (1974, p. 527). Further, he makes the link between education and modernity.

> Education itself tends to set an individual apart, especially in a predominately illiterate society. To acquire an education is also to be re-socialised into a modern western orientation in which achievement, universal, rational, criteria tend to displace ascriptive, particular and traditional norms. (Miller 1974, p. 527)

POLICYMAKING PROCESS

In terms of the policymaking process I present theories on public policymaking in Chapter 6. Policymaking is not a rational process with a beginning, a middle and an end. It should be understood as a 'chaos of purposes and accidents' (Sutton 1999, p. 5; see also Clay and Shaffer 1994; see Chapter 6). Sutton (1999) points out that concepts and tools from different disciplines can be deployed to put some order into the chaos, including policy narratives, policy communities, discourse analysis, regime theory, change management, and the role of street-level bureaucrats in implementation.

SITUATING THE ELITE THEORY AND POLICYMAKING IN MALAWI

This book focuses on the elites that implement AIDS policies. I argue AIDS policies are being produced to further the interests and agenda of national elites (Anderson 1984). However I recognise that they too are concerned about getting AIDS. Thus, that the *fisi* practice contributes significantly to the spread of HIV in Malawi is a narrative produced in line with the interests of elite groups. (The elites to which I am referring are presented in Chapter 4.) I argue that the policy making process is messy and complex and that the process of AIDS policy production in Malawi has in fact been manipulated and warped to fit in with the agendas of a small group of elites.

Studies conducted in SSA have shown a high correlation between higher education and political elite status. What the elites in my study have in common is that they all are English speaking and literate with at least secondary education and all work in some form or other on HIV and AIDS prevention. As observed by Matiki (2001) the English language is used in Malawi to provide a code, which symbolises modernisation and elitism. Elites then are likely to have a common educational background. This is an important point as in order to qualify for jobs related to HIV and development one must have to speak English and be literate. This suggests that once people use English at work and are literate they are perceived as elites as those who speak English and are literate are a minority in Malawi. However, my research demonstrates that elites in Malawi are stratified with those who have external PhDs at the top to those with degrees below them.

The elites in this study are educated thus enabling them to access employment opportunities they would not have had if they had not been educated. Further, they have adopted Christianity as their religious faith. My study demonstrates that the ideology of Christian elites within Malawi is in fact a key catalyst driving the harmful cultural practice agenda of AIDS policies.

Many scholars do separate elites into distinct groups. However, it is difficult to split the Malawian elites into groups as boundaries are fluid and often different individuals fit into multiple elite groups. For example, there is a degree of fragmentation within and between the various elites. Individuals may occupy positions within more than one elite group: a journalist may also be a religious leader or an MP may also own a private company (Lasswell and Kaplan 1950). Or a programme officer working for an AIDS NGO may also be pushing a religious agenda. Furthermore, although elites who work as AIDS officers in districts cannot be perceived as elites in the same way as urban policy makers, they are all elites.

Whereas the majority of the narratives are produced by the national elites, they are often being communicated to the general population by local elites. For example, the Church preaches through services of worship and the media that AIDS can only be controlled through abstinence and faithfulness in marriage.

The narrative of blame for AIDS is maintained that focuses on harmful cultural practices so that the elite can ensure the stability of the policy and programmes directed to reduced transmission and therefore maintain their professional status. These elites push cultural reasons over others because it makes them seem modern and also distances themselves from the crisis at a national level. As a result, they make their positions safer as they are seen as the group with which multinational agencies should engage with at a national level to solve these problems. Elites produce these narratives so they are seen as part of the solution and not part of the problem.

My argument confirms the work of Chin (2007) who stated that UNAIDS and AIDS activists accept certain myths about HIV epidemiology to keep the disease on the political agenda and, by implication, ensure funding and jobs. As Chin said 'AIDS programmes developed by international agencies and faith-based organisations have been and continue to be more socially, politically, and moralistically correct than epidemiologically accurate' (2007, p. vi). He further argues that the myth that HIV is spread easily is done either unintentionally out of genuine ignorance or misunderstanding or intentionally by deliberate exaggeration (2007, p. vi).

Epidemiology

The science of epidemiology, which includes biology, clinical medicine, social sciences and ecology, seeks to describe, understand and utilise disease patterns to improve health. Epidemiology is concerned with the spread of disease in a population. Therefore, knowing about the epidemiology of HIV is a crucial element of my theory. I draw on two decades of literature on the epidemiology of the HIV virus to determine whether the sexual practice of *fisi* contributes significantly to the spread of the disease.

Epidemiology of HIV

Key to understanding the spread of HIV (and other communicable diseases) is estimating the probability of transmission from an infected person to an uninfected one. Here, my focus is on the studies that have estimated the probability of transmission per unprotected coital act with an HIV+ partner for more than two decades, using empirical studies of serodiscordant couples (one partner is infected, the other is not) and modelling. Although such estimates cannot give the exact risk of HIV transmission for an individual, they do provide empirically based data on the *average risk of transmission*. Such estimates, according to Gray and Wawer (2012), mainly derive from empirical studies and modelling based on HIV discordant couples meaning where one partner is HIV infected and the other is not. Pilcher et al. (2004) also notes that probabilities of transmission are only derived from HIV-1 discordant couples and argues that estimates generally reflect transmission by individuals with long-term infection. Thus the data available on this topic are based on HIV discordant couples.

Transmission is much lower than is generally perceived by those living through the AIDS epidemic. In a survey conducted in Malawi, when respondents were asked what the likelihood of infection from a single act of unprotected intercourse with an infected is, over 90% said that it was 'certain' or 'highly likely' (Anglewicz 2009). The scientific literature, however, shows that it is much lower. Powers et al. (2008) conducted a review and systematic analysis of studies that produced estimates of heterosexual transmission. The analysis found that that HIV-1 transmission was commonly found to be 0.001, or 1 transmission per thousand contacts (p. 553). Findings from a study by Gray et al. (2001), also show that the overall probability of HIV transmission was 0.0011 per coital act (p. 1149). In this study, data were collected between 1994 and 1998 in a community-randomised trial of STI control of AIDS prevention in Rakai, a rural district in Uganda. 15,127 individuals aged 15–59 years were originally involved in the study and were followed up in their homes every 10 months. A subsequent study by the same researchers (Wawer et al. 2005) confirmed these results. In this study, they estimated rates of HIV-1 transmission per coital act in HIV discordant couples by stage of HIV-1 infection in the index partner and found that the overall rate of HIV transmission among discordant couples, 0.0012/coital act. Wilson et al. (2008) used the results of the Rakai 2001 study to derive a mathematical relation between viral load and the risk of HIV transmission per unprotected intercourse with an infected partner, based on a model that assumed that each sero-discordant couple had 100 sexual encounters per year. The cumulative probability of transmission to the sero-discordant partner each year was 0.0022.

Chin, a leading epidemiologist of HIV who was involved in the international response to AIDS for 20 years remarked that 'all published sex partner studies have shown that the risk of HIV transmission via sexual intercourse is a minuscule fraction of the risk associated with most other sexually transmitted diseases' (Chin 2007, p. vi).

Cofactors such as the presence of another sexually transmitted infection can decrease or increase the probability of infection, but most estimates of transmission of HIV do not take these into account

(Pilcher et al. 2004). Gray et al. (2001) highlight factors that increase the probability of infection, such as the HIV-1 viral load of the HIV-1 infected partner, younger age and genital ulceration. Their study found that transmission probabilities per coital act were highest among younger people and increased with HIV-1 viral load. Wawer et al (2005) also found higher rates of transmission during early- and late-stage infection, higher HIV load, genital ulcer disease, and younger age of the index partner. Gray et al. (2001) also found that higher infectivity in younger women could be a result of biological factors such as cervical ectopy, which might facilitate HIV-1 transmission. Assuming that some participants in the studies of HIV transmissibility had cofactors that would raise infectivity, presumably without any cofactors HIV transmission probabilities would be even lower than the average transmission probabilities cited above.

Despite factors that may increase or decrease susceptibility to HIV, transmission probabilities are low. There is no empirical research on the sexual behaviour of the male *fisi* and no evidence that this sexual practice has a higher transmission rate than other sexual practices that are common within Malawi. While a *fisi* may be more likely to be HIV positive than the average male, it is the case that intercourse with a *fisi* is usually a single act of intercourse and is far from an everyday occurrence: since intercourse within marriage is much more frequent and the use of condoms in marriage is infrequent (Chimbiri 2007), regular marital relations are thus more likely to lead to infection than one-time intercourse with a *fisi*. For HIV prevention purposes, it would be far more useful to focus on more frequent practices, such as transmission within marriages or stable couples.

During a one-off sexual act the probability of HIV-1 transmission is around 1 in 1000. Although there are factors that can increase transmission (such as genital ulcers), or decrease risk of transmission (condoms). The emphasis on eliminating the practice is due in part to the fact that accurate knowledge about the low probability of HIV has not been disseminated and, I believe, in part to the ways that policy makers and practitioners view Africans, and, since these practices are considered to be rural, the way they view rural and relatively uneducated Malawians.

My fieldwork was conducted in 2008–2009, but there is no reason to believe that there was a subsequent change in the epidemiology of HIV. If anything, the increase in reported use of condoms and the effects of antiretroviral therapy, which was just beginning to be introduced in my study period, on reducing the viral load (and thus infectiousness) of those who are HIV+, are both likely to have reduced the transmission probabilities even further.

Conclusion

In this chapter, due to the interdisciplinary nature of this research, I show how a number of theories influenced by argument. First, using the approaches used within the anthropology of development I provide a critique of HIV policy making. Second, and in order to understand how policy was constructed based on misconceptions, I draw on elite and policymaking theories to demonstrate how the policy process is being mediated by the agendas of elites as opposed to biomedical facts. Third, I use postcolonial theory to highlight how the elites are interpreting for themselves the colonial narrative that is founded on a binary opposition; civilised (the elites) and the uncivilised (the rural uneducated population) (Galtung 1971). This then enables the elites to distance themselves from those living in rural areas, allowing them to maintain a position of power and access to the resources flowing in from the aid community.

In this chapter I also review literature on HIV epidemiology. Epidemiological studies have estimated the risk of HIV-1 transmission. Although Malawians believe that HIV transmission is inevitable in a single act of unprotected intercourse (Anglewicz and Kohler 2009), epidemiologists found that the average rate of HIV transmission is 1 in 1000. These findings demonstrate that HIV is not easily transmitted. This is relevant to my study because the *fisi* practice occurs as a one-off heterosexual act and therefore it is statistically unlikely that this practice contributes significantly to the spread of HIV.

References

Anderson, J. E. (1984). *Public policymaking: An introduction* (3rd ed.). Boston, MA: Houghton Mifflin.

Anglewicz, P., & Kohler, H. P. (2009). Overestimating HIV infection: The construction and accuracy of subjective probabilities of HIV infection in rural Malawi. *Demography Research, 20*(6), 65–96.

Bassey, M. O. (1999). *Western education and political domination in Africa: A study in critical and dialogical pedagogy*. Westport, CT: Bergin and Garvey.

Bottomore, T. B. (1993). *Elites and society* (2nd ed.). New York: Routledge.

Cammack, D., McLeod, D., & Menocal, A. R., with Christiansen, K. (2006). *Donors and the 'Fragile States' agenda: A survey of current thinking and practice.* London: ODI.
Cammack, D., Golooba-Mutebi, F., Kanyongolo, F., & O'Neil, T. (2007). *Neopatrimonial politics, decentralisation and local government: Uganda and Malawi in 2006.* London: ODI.
Chabal, P., & Daloz, J. (1999). *Africa works: Disorder as political instrument.* Bloomington: Indiana University Press.
Chandra, K. (2006). What is ethnic identity and does it matter? *Annual Review of Political Science, 9*, 397–424.
Chimbiri, A. (2007). The condom is an 'intruder' in marriage: Evidence from rural Malawi. *Social Science & Medicine, 64*(5), 1102–1115.
Chin, J. (2007). *The AIDS pandemic: The collision of epidemiology with political correctness.* Oxford: Radcliffe Publishing.
Clay, E., & Shaffer, B. (Eds.). (1994). *Room for manoeuvre: An exploration of public policy in agriculture and rural development.* London: Heinemann.
Crewe, E., & Harrison, E. (1998). *Whose development? An ethnography of aid.* London: Zed.
De Waal, A. (1997). *Famine crimes: Politics and the disaster relief industry in Africa.* Oxford: James Currey.
Diop, S. (2012). African Elites and their post-colonial legacy: Cultural, political and economic discontent—By way of literature. *Africa Development, 37*(4), 221–235.
Easton, D. (1965). *A framework for political analysis.* Englewood Cliffs: Prentice Hall.
Galtung, J. (1971). A structural theory of imperialism. *Journal of Peace Research, 8*(2), 81–117.
Geo-Jaja, M. A., & Mangum, G. (2001). Structural adjustment as an inadvertent enemy of human development in Africa. *Journal of Black Studies, 32*(1), 30–49.
Gray, R. H., & Wawer, M. J. (2012). Probability of heterosexual HIV-1 transmission per coital act in Sub-Saharan Africa. *Journal of Infectious Diseases, 205* (3), 351–352.
Gray, R. H., Wawer, M. J., Brookmeyer, R., Sewankambo, N. K., Serwadda, D., Wabwire-Mangen, F., ... & Quinn, T. C. (2001). Probability of HIV-1 transmission per coital act in monogamous, heterosexual, HIV-1-discordant couples in Rakai, Uganda. *The Lancet, 357*(9263), 1149–1153.
Herrera, R. (1996). Understanding the language of politics: A study of elites and masses. *Political Science Quarterly, 111*(4), 619–637.
Higley, J., & Burton, M. (2006). *The elite foundations of liberal democracy.* Lanham: Rowman and Littlefield.

Higley, J., & Burton, M. G. (1989). The elite variable in democratic transitions and breakdowns. *American Sociological Review*, 17–32.

Hossain, N., & Moore, M. (2002). *Arguing for the poor: Elites and poverty in developing countries* (IDS Working Paper No. 148). Brighton: Institute of Development Studies.

Kitching, G. (1982). *Development and underdevelopment in historical perspective*. New York: Methuen.

Lange, S., Wallevik, H., & Kiondo, A. (2000). *Civil society in Tanzania*. Chr. Michelsen Institute.

Lasswell, H. D. (1936). *Politics: Who gets what, when, how*. Cleveland: Meridian Books.

Lasswell, H., & Kaplan, A. (1950). *Power and society New Hayen*. New Haven, CT: Yale University.

Lloyd, P. C. (1967). *Africa in social change: Changing traditional societies in the modern world*. Baltimore: Penguin Books.

Marx, K., & Engels, F. (1962). *Selected works* (Vol. II). Moscow: Foreign Languages Publishing House.

Matiki, A. J. (2001). The social significance of English in Malawi. *World Englishes, 20*(2), 201–218.

Mbeki, M. (2009). *Architects of poverty: Why Africa's capitalism needs changing*. Johannesburg: Pan Macmillan/Picador Africa.

Miller, R. A. (1974). Elite formation in Africa: Class, culture, and coherence. *The Journal of Modern African Studies, 12*(4), 521–542.

Mills, C. W. (1956). *The power elite*. NewYork: Oxford University Press.

Mosca, G. (1939 [1896]). *Elementi di scienza politica* [The ruling class]. New York: McGraw-Hill Education.

Mosse, D. (2011). Introduction: The anthropology of expertise and professionals in international development. In D. Mosse (Ed.), *Adventures in Aidland*. Oxford: Berghahn Books.

Ornett, A., & Hewitt, T. (2006). *Elites and institutions. Literature review*. Birmingham: Governance and Social Development Resource Centre, University of Birmingham.

Pareto, V. (1935 [1916]). *Trattato di Sociologia Generale* [Mind and society]. New York: Harcourt, Brace and Company.

Pilcher, C. D., Tien, H. C., Eron, J. J., Vernazza, P. L., Leu, S. Y., Stewart, P. W., ... & Cohen, M. S. (2004). Brief but efficient: Acute HIV infection and the sexual transmission of HIV. *Journal of Infectious Diseases, 189*(10), 1785–1792.

Powers, K. A., Poole, C., Pettifor, A. E., & Cohen, M. S. (2008). Rethinking the heterosexual infectivity of HIV-1: A systematic review and meta-analysis. *The Lancet Infectious Diseases, 8*, 553–563.

Sadasivam, B. (1997). The impact of structural adjustment on women: A governance and human rights agenda. *Human Rights Quarterly, 19*(3), 630–665.

Sahlins, M. (1963). Poor man, rich man, big-man, chief: Political types in Melanesia and Polynesia. *Comparative Studies in Society and History, 5*, 285–303.

Sklar, R. L. (1999). Postimperialism: Concepts and implications. *Postimperialism and World Politics, 11*.

Stiglitz, J. E. (2000). Capital market liberalization, economic growth, and instability. *World Development, 28*(6), 1075–1086.

Sutton, R. (1999). *The policy process: an overview*. London: ODI.

Svanikier, J. O. (2007). Political elite circulation: Implications for leadership diversity and democratic regime stability in Ghana. *Comparative Sociology, 6*, 114–135.

Swidler, A., & Watkins, S. C. (2009). "Teach a man to fish": The sustainability doctrine and its social consequences. *World Development, 37*(7), 1182–1196.

Van de Walle, N. (2003). Presidentialism and clientelism: Africa's emerging party systems. *Journal of Modern African Studies, 41*(2), 297–321.

Wa Thiong'o, N. (1992). *Decolonising the mind: The politics of language in African literature*. East African Publishers.

Wawer, M. J., Gray, R. H., Sewankambo, N. K., Serwadda, D., Li, X., Laeyendecker, O., et al. (2005). Rates of HIV-1 transmission per coital act, by stage of HIV-1 infection, in Rakai, Uganda. *Journal of Infectious Diseases, 191*, 1403–1409.

Whiteside, A., & Smith, J. (2009). Exceptional epidemics: AIDS still deserves a global response. *Globalization and Health, 5*(1), 15.

Wilson, D. P., Law, M. J., Grulich, A. E., Cooper, D. A., & Kaldor, J. M. (2008). Relation between HIV viral load and infectiousness: A model-based analysis. *Lancet, 372*, 314–320.

Open Access This chapter is licensed under the terms of the Creative Commons Attribution 4.0 International License (http://creativecommons.org/licenses/by/4.0/), which permits use, sharing, adaptation, distribution and reproduction in any medium or format, as long as you give appropriate credit to the original author(s) and the source, provide a link to the Creative Commons licence and indicate if changes were made.

The images or other third party material in this chapter are included in the chapter's Creative Commons licence, unless indicated otherwise in a credit line to the material. If material is not included in the chapter's Creative Commons licence and your intended use is not permitted by statutory regulation or exceeds the permitted use, you will need to obtain permission directly from the copyright holder.

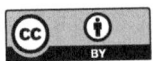

CHAPTER 3

The Development Aid Situation in Malawi

Malawi, affectionately known as the Warm Heart of Africa, is a landlocked country in sub-Saharan Africa bordered by Mozambique, Tanzania and Zambia. It is small and densely populated, with a population of 15.4 million (National Statistical Office [NSO] 2008). 85% of the population live in rural areas. Its economy is mainly dependent on agriculture, which accounts for 30% of the Gross Domestic Product. Tobacco, tea and sugar are the major export commodities (National Statistics Office and ORC Macro 2011). Malawi has three administrative regions: Northern, Central and Southern which are divided into twenty-eight districts. It has nine major ethnic groups. The national language is *Chichewa*, spoken, and English is the official language. Malawi was ruled by Britain and known as the Nyasaland protectorate from 1891 until July 1964, when Nyasaland became Malawi, and gained republic status in 1966 (National Statistics Office and ORC Macro 2011).

Despite having natural resources such as water, forests, animal life and land, according to the United Nations (UN) Malawi is one of the world's least developed countries, displaying a low Human Development Index (HDI) rating along with low socioeconomic development indicators. Its ranking on the UN's HDI is 171 out of 187 countries: 0.385, below the mean for sub-Saharan Africa of 0.389, and its per capita GNI is estimated at $911, below the mean for sub-Saharan Africa of $2050 (UN 2011). In other words, Malawi is facing devastating levels of poverty, and people are dying, which is not only reflected by official statistics but also by the number of coffin shops present on the streets of Lilongwe and Blantyre. Two-thirds of the population live below the national poverty line and more than one in five people live in ultra-poverty—unable to afford basic minimum food requirements (UN 2011).

The Aid Scene

Malawi has been receiving aid since its independence in 1964. It relies heavily on external aid. In 2011, 40% of Malawi's budget came from foreign donors (Donnelly 2011). And between 2007 and 2009 aid contributed approximately a fifth of the country's GNI (World Bank 2011). In 2008 Malawi received close to US$1 billion in official development aid including from Britain, Japan, the USA, the IMF, the World Bank (Myroniuk 2011). Despite this aid dependency, Malawi experienced rapid growth between 2005 and 2010 and its economy grew at an average of 7%. The World Bank credited this growth to 'sound economic policies and a supportive donor environment' (World Bank 2013).

When the former President Bingu wa Mutharika and his Democratic Progressive Party won a landslide second term in the May 2009 elections it was seen as a remuneration for their success since their first election victory in 2004. However, from 2010 Malawi's economic growth began to slow (Wroe 2012). According to the World Bank this was due to a deterioration in the policy environment (World Bank 2013). This resulted in foreign exchange, fuel and electricity supply shortages and the cost of living kept going up.

In the late 1970s the International Monetary Fund and the World Bank offered financial assistance to countries in the Global South while applying a neoliberal economic ideology as a precondition to receiving the funds. Many countries in sub-Saharan Africa accepted the economic liberalisation measures and introduced rigorous structural adjustment policy reforms. Malawi was one such country. In 1979, with support from both institutions, and in response to a declining macroeconomic situation, the Malawi Government implemented economic stabilisation and structural reforms (Conroy et al. 2006). The IMF stabilisation policies aimed at restoring external sector balances through exchange rate management reforms and balance of payment support through Stabilisation Adjustment Loans (SALs). The World Bank provided development and reconstruction funds through Structural Adjustment

Policies (SAPs) and Fiscal Restructuring and Deregulation Programmes (FRDP).

These structural reforms were adopted in an attempt to liberalise the economy, broaden and diversify the production base, and allocate resources more productively (Munthali 2004). Although the specifics of SAPs differ, four basic elements were always present: currency devaluation, the removal/reduction of the state from the workings of the economy, the elimination of subsidies to reduce expenditures, and trade liberalisation. Such prerequisites were intended to lead to the adjustment of malfunctioning economies in order to become viable components of a global system (Riddel 1992).

The IMF and World Bank argued that such reforms would reduce poverty. However, this model of development, whereby the North imposed conditions on the South, came under attack: programmes of the IMF and the World Bank in fact increase poverty. The ideology of neoliberalism required poor countries to reduce spending on social issues including health, education and development, while debt repayment and other economic policies prioritised (Sadasivam 1997; Geo-Jaja and Mangum 2001). Evidence shows that neglect and underfunding of the social sector particularly education and health, negate the development of a skilled labour pool, the capacity and capability build-up in research and policy, and the provision of the management talents demanded in an adjusting economy. As Stiglitz points out:

> The IMF likes to go about its business without outsiders asking too many questions. In theory, the fund supports democratic institutions in the nations it assists. In practice, it undermines the democratic process by imposing policies. Officially, of course, the IMF doesn't 'impose' anything. It 'negotiates' the conditions for receiving aid. But all the power in the negotiations is on one side—the IMF's—and the fund rarely allows sufficient time for broad consensus-building or even widespread consultations with either parliaments or civil society. Sometimes the IMF dispenses with the pretence of openness altogether and negotiates secret covenants. (Stiglitz 2000, p. 56)

One report critical of World Bank conditionality produced by the Dutch NGO A SEED was based on desk research from country case studies including Malawi, Mali, Mozambique, Nicaragua, Zambia and Bangladesh. The report concluded that privatisation and liberalisation policies that are neither designed, nor desired by countries, are still pushed through by the World Bank; it also reported that the implementation of World Bank promoted policies correlated with an increase in levels of poverty. The report called for the Dutch government to demand a phase out of economic policy conditionality, which would have brought it in line with other European governments, including the UK and Norway (Cabello et al. 2008).

The IMF in 1999 replaced Structural Adjustment Programmes (SAPs) with Poverty Reduction Growth Facility (PRGF) and Policy Framework Papers with Poverty Reduction Strategy Papers (PSRP) as the policy framework for determining loan and debt relief. PRSPs set out a country's macroeconomic, structural and social policies to improve growth rates and reduce poverty. Such strategies for reform were necessary for World Bank loans or lending by the IMF under the poverty reduction and growth facility. However, many critics uphold the view that the PRSPs are as equally detrimental as the SAPs. Countries still have to fulfil donor criteria; therefore, aid is still tied to conditionalities. Further, they did not incorporate gender, race and poverty interests (Bretton Woods 2004).

The Millennium Development Goals (MDGs) were also a further initiative to reduce poverty. Economic growth rates were not considered part of the MDGs, however there is widespread agreement that the MDGs placed poverty reduction at the centre of the development agenda at least in international discussions and policy discourse (Watkins 2011). At the Millennium Summit in September 2000, the largest gathering of world leaders in history adopted the UN Millennium Declaration, committing to reduce extreme poverty and setting time-bound targets, with a deadline of 2015. The MDGs were the world's time-bound and quantified targets for addressing extreme poverty in its many dimensions—income, poverty, hunger, disease, lack of adequate shelter, and exclusion—while promoting gender equality, education and environmental sustainability. They were also basic human rights— the rights of each person on the planet to health, education, shelter and security. The purpose of the MDGs was not to change thinking but to change policies and outcomes. They were designed to 'encourage sustainable pro-poor development progress and donor support of domestic efforts in this direction' (Manning 2009, p. 19).

Critics of the MDGs say they were cobbled together in order to make politicians look grand for the UN Millennium Declaration and targets were set in the absence of any idea of how they were going to be met, how much it would cost, or where the money was coming from. The 'one size fits all' target percentage reductions mean that countries that have achieved a lot in the past have big difficulties in meeting the goals, and gains (or lack of them) took no account of distribution across socioeconomic groupings and that they are a factor in the rise of disease specific global programmes instead of sector-wide reforms. A further criticism of the MDGs is that they did not track misconceptions concerning the HIV virus. As England said: 'We will not achieve better health care for the world's poor without better national health systems to fund and deliver it, and we will not achieve that without a better international system for aid' (England 2007, p. 565).

Malawi adopted an MDG-focused national plan to reduce poverty called the Malawi Growth and Development Strategy (MGDS) (2006–2011) (Kenny and Summer 2011). The MGDS addressed six thematic areas which were sustainable economic growth; social protection; social development; management and prevention of nutrition disorders and HIV/AIDS; infrastructure development; and improved governance. Despite developing a 'home-grown overarching national policy for creating new wealth, for achieving sustainable economic growth and development and for combating endemic poverty' (GoM 2007, p. 2) the former President, Bingu wa Mutharika, faced a strict set of aid conditionalities to disburse the US$5.3 billion in foreign aid received between 2004 and 2011 (World Bank 2011). He had to run the Malawian economy along guidelines set out by the IMF, abide by various UN agreements, and adhere to Malawi's constitutional framework.

Under his rule Malawi faced serious problems with international donors. In November 2009, he accused the World Bank and the IMF with causing foreign exchange shortages by forcing the country to liberalise the economy. Throughout 2010, the IMF pressured the administration to devalue the Malawi Kwacha in order to encourage investment and trade but the government ignored the advice. The IMF took the unusual step of asking a group of donors to release their budget support grants to Malawi, which they had been withholding until a new IMF programme was approved. The IMF board shifted the decision for a new programme for Malawi to mid-February, raising fears that donors would continue to withhold $545 million in aid.

International donors became increasingly concerned with the government's failure to devalue the currency and its repeated unconstitutional behaviour, including the stifling of opponents, refusal of holding local elections and Mutharika spending eight million pounds on a private jet. This was expressed when a group called the Common Approach to Budgetary Support group (CABS), including Malawi's two biggest donors (the EU and DFID), called a meeting with the government in March 2011. The group announced that it was suspending aid and that it would permanently withdraw budgetary support if the government failed to address its concerns. A leaked document from the British High Commissioner demonstrated more explicitly why donors were worried. The Commissioner, Fergus Cochrane-Dyet, described Mutharika as 'becoming ever more autocratic and intolerant of criticism' (*The Guardian* 2011). The document indicated the willingness of the British government to suspend aid if the state of affairs persisted. When the document came to light in April, the government promptly expelled the diplomat from the country and Britain responded by announcing that it would review all of its ongoing financial support to the Malawian government.

The UK Department for International Development, then Malawi's largest bilateral donor with US$121 million donated per year, of which $49 million went to funding Malawi's public health sector, made its final aid disbursement to the country in March 2011, and decided not to renew a six-year spending commitment. Other development partners decided to end or suspend general budget support to Malawi (The World Bank, The EU, The African Development Bank, Germany and Norway) (Tran 2011), or tried to force change on a host of issues, including Malawi's enforcement of an anti-homosexuality law and government threats to freedom of speech and association. The World Bank withheld $40 million in funding, Germany suspended $16.5 million, because of the anti-gay laws ns the Global Fund to Fight AIDS, Tuberculosis and Malaria (GFTAM) rejected a $565 million plan (Donnelly 2011).

Following on from the Common Approach to Budgetary Support meeting Mutharika attacked Malawi's donors in a widely reported speech. He accused them of siding with civil society organisations against the government and claimed that, as he was Malawi's leader, donors should privilege their relationship with him. Mutharika's speech did not directly address the concerns raised by donors, referring to them only as 'lies' spread by civil society groups. Donors' decisions to withhold funds had a detrimental impact on Malawi's economy and healthcare system as Malawi's health sector is nearly entirely donor funded. With foreign aid covering about 90% of the cost of all medicines in Malawi, drug stock-outs became more common and physicians frustrated they were unable to prescribe medicines, leading to low morale, IRIN (2011) notes. Mutharika stated that Malawi should become far less dependent on donors, despite its reliance on donor aid, which helped lead to substantial gains, including putting 270,000 people on antiretroviral treatment since 2004 (Donnelly 2011). Mutharika, however, praised China for its unconditional aid and said that China did not demand democratic reforms, good governance and anti-corruption drives as a condition for aid and trade.

In this section I have set the development aid scene in Malawi and demonstrated the powerful and influential role international donors play in influencing policy and programmes. I have shown how aid conditionality can lead to failed projects. I have also demonstrated how funding is donor led and if donors are not happy with what is happening in the country to which they are supplying aid, whether it is the way money is being spent, or the type of policies the government implements, then funding will be withdrawn. It further illustrates how donor policies do not take into account in-country situations and make their own conditions for the release of funds. In all these points made above I make a case that international aid is linked to conditions that often are not evidence-based but based on the perceptions highlighted by the Malawian elites. Further it shows that funding flows from donors can often be volatile and reflect priorities that are not shared by national governments. The next section looks at AIDS in Malawi.

AIDS

UNAIDS, the joint United Nations programme on HIV/AIDS, was established in 1996 in an attempt to coordinate efforts to curb the pandemic. At the first ever Special Session on HIV/AIDS of the United Nations General Assembly (UNGASS) in 2001, UN Member States endorsed the *Declaration of Commitment on HIV/AIDS to address MDG 6*. This *Declaration* included time-bound pledges to generate measurable action and concrete progress in the AIDS response. Signed by 189 world leaders, the Declaration agreed that HIV/AIDS was a national and international development issue of the highest priority (UNAIDS 2006). This signed declaration led to increased funding for international

HIV/AIDS programmes. At the five-year review of implementation of the *Declaration of Commitment* in 2006, UN Member States reaffirmed the pledges made at the 2001 Special Session. In the *Political Declaration on HIV/AIDS*, Member states committed to taking action to move towards universal access to HIV prevention, treatment, care and support by 2010 (UNAIDS 2008).

Given the above, it has been argued that AIDS had become not just a health priority but a global development priority. This can be seen in the case of Malawi. The *National HIV/AIDS Policy* (2003) in its preamble summarises the impact of HIV/AIDS as:

- A public health issue because it directly affects the health of large numbers of people in society and reduces the overall health status and well being of the nation.
- A social issue because it adversely impacts families and communities resulting in excessive medical expenses, depleted family savings and leading to disposal of assets.
- An economic issue because it leads to a decline in economic growth, by reducing the productivity of the labour force.
- Development issues because it is weakening institutions and destroying institutional memory in both the public and private sectors—destroying their capacity to formulate, analyse and manage public policies, and develop programmes and strategies essential for economic growth. (Malawi, & Malawi. National AIDS Commission 2003, pp. 2–3)

UNAIDS was created because the epidemic was considered to be exceptional, thus requiring exceptional efforts at prevention and mitigation. That HIV requires a response above 'normal' health interventions began as a Western response to the virus (Smith and Whiteside 2010) and the international community has also said it was exceptional (Dionne et al. 2013). AIDS exceptionalists emphasise the importance of human rights issues in relation to AIDS. Those against exceptionalism, and particularly well-known, is England, who holds the view that funding for health systems and funding for HIV amounts to a zero-sum game: 'until we put HIV in its place, countries will not get the delivery systems they need' (England 2007, p. 1073). In other words, the HIV pandemic stimulated an exceptional response.

According to UNAIDS figures in 2007 an estimated 33 million people were infected with HIV worldwide of which 2.5 million people were newly infected and there were 2.1 million AIDS-related deaths (UNAIDS 2007). Southern Africa is the area hardest hit by the pandemic, accounting for 68% of the global population living with HIV and almost 32% of all new HIV infections and AIDS-related deaths globally. It is projected that by 2015 more than 45 million people will have died from AIDS-related illnesses globally. A further 200 million people will be directly affected, based on conservative estimates that only 1 in 5 members of the family will be affected by each person who dies, and an additional 200 million people will be less directly affected (Poku 2005). However, the long-term impact of AIDS is hard to measure, because there is a differential impact over time as an infected individual's health deteriorates, and a time lag between infection and death (Poku 2004).

Malawi's National HIV Policy and Sexual Cultural Practices

In Malawi, the government's national HIV policy stipulates that: 'many practices, including polygamy, extramarital relations and customary practices such as widow and widower inheritance, death cleansing, forced sex for young girls coming of age (*fisi*) increase the risk of HIV infection' (Malawi, & Malawi. National AIDS Commission 2003, p. 24). Practices exist that are perceived as culturally acceptable but said to spread HIV by legitimising high-risk behaviour. These include *chokolo* (widow inheritance), *nthena* (widower given wife's younger sister in the Northern region) widow cleansing, *m'bvade* (unmarried female's post-natal abstinence is concluded by surrogate sex), the use of *fisi* (surrogate) in male fertility in most ethnic groups; the use of *fisi* in initiation rites among the Yao; and the belief that STIs, including HIV, can be prevented by charms and 'vaccines' (Lwanda 2005, p. 125). Powerful and pervasive beliefs and practices, based on deep-rooted associations between sex, health, and illness, continue to influence sexual and reproductive health and health-seeking behaviour. However, given the secrecy that surrounds beliefs and practices which are linked to fertility, plus the many variations from village to village, it is very difficult to be specific about the extent to which these practices are continuing to take place or where they take place (P26, P37) which makes the link between them and HIV transmission more tenuous. I will now describe the following practices: polygamy, *fisi* and widow inheritance.

Polygamy has been identified by the Government of Malawi as accelerating the spread of HIV. If one partner is infected within a polygamous family the number of persons at risk becomes higher than in a monogamous family. But it is not polygamy itself that spreads HIV but the practice of unsafe sex. A polygamous family in which all partners practise safe sex in their extramarital affairs is no more at risk than a monogamous family, particularly given that men in a so-called monogamous relationship may still be having affairs. Therefore, what is important is not polygamy or monogamy but the practice of safe sex in extramarital relationships. Fighting against polygamy will not make people practise safe sex. Polygamy is deeply ingrained in a number of African countries, and is part of a complex set of social and economic relations, which means it is unlikely that the practice could be eradicated. According to Jacoby (1995) there is 'polygamy belt' stretching across Africa, from Senegal to Tanzania. Despite the extensive polygamy discourse, monogamy dominates in Malawi. The extent of polygamy in Malawi was measured in the 2004 Malawi Demographic Health Survey. Overall 84% of all currently married women are in monogamous unions, 12% are in polygamous unions with one cowife and 3% are in polygamous unions with two or more cowives. These statistics demonstrate that only a small percentage of women are in polygamous unions. This raises questions why the Government of Malawi is concentrating on changing this practice as a root trigger of AIDS.

Widow inheritance is also cited in Malawi's HIV policy as a practice that contributes to the spread of HIV. Widow inheritance is a practice whereby widows are 'inherited' by a male family member of her late husband, often the brother. It was initially designed as an economic relationship, so that the wife and her children could continue to be supported by the deceased husband's brother. Since it is believed that the brother who died must have died of AIDS, the practice came to be considered a risk factor in HIV transmission. According to Swidler and Watkins (2009) it is unlikely that widow inheritance does much to transmit HIV: rather, it is transmitted through marriage or extramarital partnerships. Here it is important to note again that the probability of transmission of HIV in a single act of unprotected intercourse is very low—1 in 1000 (.001) if there are no current STIs or ulcers and if the sex occurs outside the brief window period or at the end, when viral load is high. Even if there are other risk factors the risk increases to 8 in 1000 (.008), still low.

Thus, the probability of the virus being passed on from the brother to the widow or vice versa is very low. However, if the widow or the brother had contracted HIV before the widow inheritance practice took place then if unprotected sex is carried out the probability of contracting the virus can increase. As Lwanda (2005) points out he noted five examples of educated Christian men who had inherited their relatives' widows with tragic results. There were clear signs and symptoms suggestive of AIDS in all cases. Again it is not so much the practice that is conducive to the spread of HIV but the practice and negotiation of safe sex.

Fisi is also described in Malawi's HIV policy as a practice which contributes to the spread of HIV during initiation ceremonies. Initiation ceremonies celebrate the transition to adulthood, and in that sense are equivalent to a Bar Mitzvah or a Latin American Quinceanera festivity. In Malawi, traditional initiation counsellors typically provide information on the expected conduct of the initiates, both male and female, when they become an adult. Initiation ceremonies are far more frequently celebrated for girls than for boys. At initiation, girls who have started menstruating are separated from those who have not. They are advised to 'avoid' male friends because of the risk of pregnancy and sexually transmitted infections. Some respondents told me that girls are taught how to respond to future husbands when having sex, although secrecy prevented them from telling me more. However, rapid external societal changes have taken place, which have brought about changes to the nature of some rituals. For example, traditionally, when a girl and boy who had reached puberty were accepted as 'girlfriend and boyfriend', the closing of the initiation ceremony would present the opportunity for them to consummate the relationship. As such, they then reached adulthood as a married couple. Yet there is a dearth of data exploring the impact of initiation ceremonies on young people in sub-Saharan Africa.

Among some societies in Malawi and Zambia (Moyo and Müller 2011) a man is hired as a *fisi* (hyena) to have sex with the female initiates. One explanation for such a practice may be that the introduction of formal education schedules has resulted in girls being initiated at a younger age, and before they are considered ready for marriage. According to Coombes (2001), such rituals are said to increase exposure to STI/HIV and pregnancy, and undermine the human rights of children, and their ability to recognise and resist sexual abuse.

Views on Culture

Cultural norms are widely held in Malawi that women should be inexperienced and naive in sexual matters and that pleasing men is the primary goal of sex (P7, P26). From very young ages, girls are treated as sexual beings whose primary objective is to please men, while boys are never taught what it takes to please a woman sexually. A review of cultural beliefs and practices influencing sexual and reproductive health and health-seeking behaviour (Matinga and McConville 2003) found that, as in other countries in the region, the main risk factor concerning sexual and reproductive health in Malawi is that 'being a man' means being dominant and in control, particularly in sexual liaisons. Females who want acceptance in society are expected to be meek, and sexually submissive to the point where it is not acceptable to say 'no' to sex (Coombes 2001). This may reflect the fact that whereas Malawi's complex history has resulted in the coexistence of both matrilineal and patrilineal kinship systems, both are strongly patriarchal (i.e. power lies with the male members of the family). The belief in the 'powerlessness' of females in sexual decision-making continues to place both women and men—young or old, married or unmarried—at great risk.

The following is an excerpt from my journal notes.

> Angela is currently working as a consultant employed by UNDP. She is working with the Ministry of Agriculture on a communications strategy. She and I talked over lunch about relationships. Angela is from Uganda. We talked about African men. She said African men are the same wherever you are. They have extramarital affairs and they perceive having more than one woman as moving up the social ladder. She told me her husband had an affair and she did not find out until she was informed that one of the children had died. But not her child, the child her husband had fathered with another woman. Angela is still married to him and I asked why? Why have you not divorced him? She said that in Africa it is difficult to divorce your husband. It is frowned upon – a type of social stigma is attached to divorce. She explained that if she were to divorce her husband then everything she has achieved in her life would mean nothing. (Journal entry, 7 February 2009)

This conversation highlights how male promiscuity is problematic for women: it locks them into relationships in which their sexual behaviour is highly controlled through views of modesty. They are vulnerable to infection by a construction of masculine sexuality that pursues promiscuity. This reality again contests the argument that prevalence is higher in rural communities that carry out harmful cultural practices. Women's weak societal position and practices that remove choice from them compound gender imbalance (Geisler 1997, p. 92). For example, men offering to pay more money to sleep with sex workers without a condom. This male dominance extends to exposing elite women to STIs through the sexual behaviour of their men who have mistresses. Thus, high socioeconomic status is, in Malawi, a risk factor for HIV infection. Higher HIV prevalence rates are found among women in the highest wealth quintile than the lowest. Further, women with a secondary or more than secondary education have higher HIV prevalence rates than women with no education (MDHS 2010).

The societal norms that enable men to engage in multiple sexual relationships both before and after marriage are manifested in extramarital relationships, divorce and marriage-remarriage cycles. One person told me 'there is this belief that for you to be recognised as a man in the society you have to have multiple partners' (P42). Another said 'men take pleasure in having multiple sexual partners' (P41). Women perceive that they are at risk because their husbands have unprotected sex with other partners and because women are much less likely to engage in higher-risk sex than men (MDHS, survey 2005, p. 201). Men perceive that the risks they face arise from having unprotected sex with other partners.

I interviewed a lawyer who has a Ph.D. She told me:

> It's normal for men to have multiple sexual partners but not because that is a cultural practice, no, that is an issue of behaviour. But you see that issue of behaviour is very much influenced by our culture. And hence, we all know worldwide that HIV/AIDS is fuelled by multiple sexual partners, especially in cases where people are not resorting to protected sex. And that is the case in Malawi. Another link that you can see between the influences of our culture on HIV/AIDS spread is that women tend to take a subordinate role in society, usually they are voiceless. So you find that in cases where a man and a woman want to engage in sexual intercourse, you find that the woman is so powerless; as a matter of fact you don't question what a man wants to do, especially for the rural folk. They will never demand for protected sex, they never bargain for things like condoms. There are a number of factors that contribute to this; the economic factors, because women are trading sex for money and that leaves you at a very bargaining point; the cultural practices that have employed us as women

> not to question the ways of our husbands for instance. so you find that in the many family set up the women cannot say to their husbands that you know what I think lets go without sex because I don't know if you've been handling yourself right, No, ok but can we please have protected sex. But, what is the case to me is that our culture has influenced our behaviour, where the man is superior the woman is subordinate, where it is the sign of masculine power to have as many sexual partners as you can, and where it is actually law as custom for a man to have as many wives as possible, and you see how that can really offer a very environment for the transmission of HIV/AIDS coupled with of course other factors. When you look at the issue of HIV/AIDS, mind you, I like a holistic approach to the factors that fuel it because they work so much in complementation of each other, you can never isolate culture as a separate factor, you see that also the economic factors come in because if the women were empowered economically then maybe this whole question of men having multiple sexual partners would have died a natural death because sometimes you are forced to be in the polygamous arrangement because you want to benefit economically. So, when you go try and also explore how these other factors are complementing. The dual system of the law that we have at the moment, I know if you go back to the law commission they will tell you that they've tried to consolidate our marriage laws into one act, and maybe you may wish to explore how they have tackled this issue that for as long as that legislation remains the bill the situation at the moment is that our law recognises marriages that are constructed under the marriage act that's strictly polygamous marriages, then it recognises marriages that are constructed under the Christian rights act and customary marriages, which are potentially polygamous; and which, unfortunately, so many of us are governed by. Even myself, I constructed a religious marriage, I went to my church, the Roman Catholic Church; but at the end of the day that's not a marriage under the marriage act. If my husband were to choose to have another wife, he could. (P26)

I interviewed a Cabinet Minister who has a Ph.D. She told me:

> A real man must propose a woman because a woman does not propose a man. So the traditional practice is that you wait for a man to propose you and therefore men take pleasure in having multiple sexual partners and they are known as these are the real men. On the other hand women feel they have to be proposed. That's a sign that you are beautiful. If nobody proposes you, you must be an ugly woman. So those are parts of the social cultural practices that are taking place. While on the other hand traditionally you are initiated not to say no to sexual intercourse because if

you say no you are sending the man to another woman and you lose out. Especially in marriage and therefore women have no power to negotiate for safer sexual intercourse. So you have that dilemma. And women are expected to be faithful while it is ok for men to be promiscuous. So there is an imbalance. So these are some of the cultural practices that are out there. (P41)

Conclusion

In this chapter I have set the development aid scene in Malawi and demonstrated the powerful and influential role international donors play in influencing policy and programmes. I have shown how aid conditionality can lead to failed projects. I have also demonstrated how funding is donor led and if donors are not happy with what is happening in the country to which they are supplying aid, whether it is the way money is being spent, or the type of policies the government implements, then funding will be withdrawn. It further illustrates how donor policies do not take into account in-country situations and make their own conditions for the release of funds. In all these points made above I make a case that international aid is linked to conditions that often are not evidence-based but based on the perceptions highlighted by the Malawian elites. Further it shows that funding flows from donors can often be volatile and reflect priorities that are not shared by national governments.

References

Bretton Woods. (2004). Retrieved January 14, 2012, from http://www.brettonwoodsproject.org/art.shtml?x=42231.

Cabello, D., Sekulova, F., & Schmidt, D. (2008). *World Bank conditionalities: Poor deal for poor countries.* Amsterdam, The Netherlands: A SEED Europe.

Conroy, A., Blackie, M., Whiteside, A., Malewezi, J., & Sachs, J. (2006). *Poverty, AIDS and hunger: Breaking the poverty trap in Malawi.* Hampshire: Palgrave Macmillan.

Coombes, Y. (2001). *A literature review to support the situational analysis for the national behaviour change interventions strategy on HIV/AIDS and sexual and reproductive health.* London: DFID.

Dionne, K. Y., Gerland, P., & Watkins, S. C. (2013). Aids exceptionalism: Another constituency heard from. *AIDS and Behavior, 17*(3), 825–831.

Donnelly, J. (2011). Battles with donors cloud Malawi's HIV prevention plan. *The Lancet, 378*(9787), 215–216.

England, R. (2007). The dangers of disease specific aid programmes. *British Medical Journal, 335,* 565.

Geisler, G. (1997). Women are women or how to please your husband: Initiation ceremonies and the politics of 'Tradition' in Southern Africa. *African Anthropology, 14*(1), 92–128.

Geo-Jaja, M. A., & Mangum, G. (2001). Structural adjustment as an inadvertent enemy of human development in Africa. *Journal of Black Studies, 32*(1), 30–49.

Malawi, & Malawi. National AIDS Commission. (2003). National HIV/AIDS Policy: A Call to Renewed Action (Vol. 2). Office of the President and Cabinet, National AIDS Commission.

Government of Malawi. (2007). *Malawi and the millennium development goals.* Lilongwe, Malawi: Government of Malawi.

IRIN. (2011). MALAWI: UK aid cuts hit health care. Retrieved June 6, 2011, from http://www.irinnews.org/report/92877/malawi-uk-aid-cuts-hit-health-care.

Jacoby, H. G. (1995). The economics of polygyny in sub-Saharan Africa: Female productivity and the demand for wives in Côte d'Ivoire. *Journal of Political Economy, 103*(5), 938–971.

Kenny, C., & Summer, A. (2011). *More money or more development: What have the MDGs achieved?* Washington, DC: Centre for Global Development.

Lwanda, J. (2005). *Politics, culture and medicine in Malawi.* Zomba: Kachere.

Macro, O. R. C. (2005). *Malawi demographic and health survey 2004.* Zomba, Malawi: National Statistical Office.

Manning, R. (2009). *Using indicators to encourage development: Learning lessons from the millennium development goals* (No. 2009: 01). Danish Institute for International Studies.

Matinga, P., & McConville, F. (2003). *A review of cultural beliefs and practices influencing sexual and reproductive health and health-seeking behaviour, in Malawi.* Lilongwe: Department for International Development Malawi (DFID).

Moyo, N., & Müller, J. C. (2011). The influence of cultural practices on the HIV and AIDS pandemic in Zambia. *HTS Theological Studies, 67*(3), 412–417.

Munthali, T. (2004). *The impact of Structural Adjustment Policies (SAPs) on manufacturing growth in Malawi* (No. 0410002). EconWPA.

Myroniuk, T. W. (2011). Global discourses and experiential speculation: Secondary and tertiary graduate Malawians dissect the HIV/AIDS epidemic. *Journal of the International AIDS Society, 14*(1), 47.

NSO. (2008). *Multiple indicator cluster survey.* Zomba: National Statistical Office.

NSO, M., & Macro, I. C. F. (2011). *Malawi demographic and health survey 2010.* Zomba, Malawi and Calverton, MD: NSO and ORC Macro.

Poku, N. K. (2005). *AIDS in Africa: How the poor are dying.* Cambridge, UK: Polity Press.

Poku, N. K., & Whiteside, A. (2004). Introduction: Africa's HIV/AIDS crisis. In N. K. Poku & A. Whiteside (Eds.), *The political economy of AIDS in Africa* (pp. xvii–xxii). Hampshire, UK: Ashgate.

Riddel, J. B. (1992). Things fall apart again: Structural adjustment programmes in sub-Saharan Africa. *The Journal of Modern African Studies, 30*(1), 53–68.

Sadasivam, B. (1997). The impact of structural adjustment on women: A governance and human rights agenda. *Human Rights Quarterly, 19*(3), 630–665.

Smith, J. H., & Whiteside, A. (2010). The history of AIDS exceptionalism. *Journal of the International AIDS Society, 13*(1), 47.

Stiglitz, J. (2000). What I learned at the world economic crisis. *Globalization and the poor: Exploitation or equalizer,* 195–204.

Swidler, A., & Watkins, S. (2009). "Teach a man to fish": The sustainability doctrine and its social consequences. *World Development, 37*(7), 1182–1196.

The Guardian. (2011). Britain expels Malawi ambassador in retaliation after envoy is ordered out. Retrieved June 14, 2011, from http://www.theguardian.com/world/2011/apr/27/britain-malawi-ambassador-expelled?INTCMP=SRCH.

Tran, M. (2011). Britain suspends aid to Malawi. Retrieved July 14, 2011, from http://www.guardian.co.uk/global-development/2011/jul/14/britain-suspends-aid-to-malawi.

UN. (2011). *One plan annual report: United Nations Country Team.* Lilongwe, Malawi: UN.

UNAIDS. (2006). *2006 report on the global AIDS epidemic.* Geneva, Switzerland: UNAIDS.

UNAIDS. (2007). *Practical guidelines for intensifying HIV prevention, towards universal access.* Geneva, Switzerland: UNAIDS.

UNAIDS. (2008). *2008 report on the global AIDS epidemic.* Geneva, Switzerland: UNAIDS.

Watkins, K. (2011). The millennium development goals: Three proposals for renewing the vision and reshaping the future. Retrieved October 10, 2013, from http://www.scribd.com/doc/2442520/Millennium-Development-Goals.

World Bank. (2011). *Global monitoring report 2011: Improving the odds of achieving the MDGs.* Washington, DC: World Bank.

World Bank. (2013). *Malawi overview.* Retrieved October 6, 2013, from http://www.worldbank.org/en/country/malawi/overview.

Wroe, D. (2012). Donors, dependency, and political crisis in Malawi. *African Affairs, 111*(442), 135–144.

Young, J., & Mendizabal, E. (2009). An anthropological critique of development: The growth of ignorance, volume 53 of ODI briefing paper. London: Overseas Development Institute.

Open Access This chapter is licensed under the terms of the Creative Commons Attribution 4.0 International License (http://creativecommons.org/licenses/by/4.0/), which permits use, sharing, adaptation, distribution and reproduction in any medium or format, as long as you give appropriate credit to the original author(s) and the source, provide a link to the Creative Commons licence and indicate if changes were made.

The images or other third party material in this chapter are included in the chapter's Creative Commons licence, unless indicated otherwise in a credit line to the material. If material is not included in the chapter's Creative Commons licence and your intended use is not permitted by statutory regulation or exceeds the permitted use, you will need to obtain permission directly from the copyright holder.

CHAPTER 4

'Harmful Cultural Practices' and AIDS

GLOBAL POLICIES ON GENDER-BASED VIOLENCE, AIDS AND HARMFUL CULTURAL PRACTICES

The UN Secretary General highlighted in a report in 2012 that 'the Political Declaration on HIV/AIDS recognised the harmful effects of unequal gender norms and practices and pledged concerted action to eliminate gender inequalities' (UN 2012, p. 19). In the 2011 UN Political Declaration on HIV and AIDS: Intensifying our efforts to eliminate HIV and AIDS (UN 2011) member states agreed to 'pledge to eliminate gender inequalities and gender-based abuse and violence, increase the capacity of women and adolescent girls to protect themselves from the risk of HIV infection' (UN 2011, p. 8). This policy suggests that, in order for women to reduce the risk of contracting HIV, gender-based violence needs to be addressed. Although this declaration does not name specific harmful cultural practices, it mentions the 'harmful effects of unequal gender norms and practices' (UN 2011, p. 9).

In its resolution 2003/45 of 23 April 2003, on the elimination of violence against women, the Commission on Human Rights affirmed that the term 'violence against women' meant any act of gender-based violence that resulted in, or was likely to result in, physical, sexual or psychological harm or suffering to women, including, among others, crimes committed in the name of honour, and traditional practices

© The Author(s) 2019
S. Page, *Development, Sexual Cultural Practices and HIV/AIDS in Africa*, https://doi.org/10.1007/978-3-030-04119-9_4

harmful to women, including female genital mutilation, early and forced marriages, female infanticide and dowry-related violence and deaths. It strongly condemned such violence. It emphasised that violence against women and girls, including female genital mutilation and early and forced marriage, could increase their vulnerability to HIV infection. The Commission called upon states to condemn violence against women and girls and not to invoke custom, tradition or practices in the name of religion or culture to avoid their obligations to eliminate such violence.

In this resolution we see that the terms or categories of violence against women and gender-based violence have both been adopted. We also see that specific practices are listed that are deemed harmful to women with the suggestion that these practices may increase women's vulnerability to HIV/AIDS. This resolution is more detailed than the political declaration on HIV/AIDS and calls on member states to condemn violence against women and not to invoke 'custom, tradition or practices in the name of religion or culture to avoid their obligations to eliminate such violence' (UN Commission on Human Rights 2003, p. 4). These global policies show how cultural practices, gender-based violence and AIDS emerged as key development priorities. The UN General Assembly in its January 2002 Resolution on Traditional or Customary Practices affecting the health of women and girls called upon all states to ratify or accede to the Committee on the Elimination of Discrimination against Women (CEDAW), and to adopt national measures to prohibit traditional practices.

The emergence of harmful cultural practices in global development conventions and policies came about at the 1993 World Conference on Human Rights. The UN Declaration on the Elimination of Violence Against Women (UN 1993) made the link between gender-based violence and harmful cultural practices and defined violence against women as 'any act of gender-based violence that results in or is likely to result in physical, sexual or psychological harm or suffering to women' (UN 1993, p. 1). Under article 2 it stipulated that violence against women should be understood as:

> (a) Physical, sexual and psychological violence occurring in the family, including battering, sexual abuse of female children in the household, dowry-related violence, marital rape, female genital mutilation and other traditional practices harmful to women, non-spousal violence and violence

related to exploitation; (b) Physical, sexual and psychological violence occurring within the general community, including rape, sexual abuse, sexual harassment and intimidation at work, in educational institutions and elsewhere, trafficking in women and forced prostitution; and (c) Physical, sexual and psychological violence perpetrated or condoned by the State, wherever it occurs. (p. 2)

On 7 February 2000 resolution A/RES/54/133 was adopted by the UN General Assembly: 'Traditional or customary practices affecting the health of women and girls'. The resolution:

> Emphasises the need for technical and financial assistance to developing countries working to achieve the elimination of traditional or customary practices affecting the health of women and girls from United Nations funds and programmes, international and regional financial institutions and bilateral and multilateral donors, as well as the need for assistance to non-governmental organisations and community-based groups active in this field from the international community. (UN 2000, p. 4)

In other words, international donors are encouraged to provide technical and financial assistance to developing countries to eliminating traditional practices because they affect women's and girls health. Second, it called upon member states:

(a) To ratify or accede to, if they have not yet done so, the relevant human rights treaties, in particular the Convention on the Elimination of All Forms of Discrimination against Women and the Convention on the Rights of the Child, and to respect and implement fully their obligations under any such treaties to which they are parties;

(b) To implement their international commitments in this field, inter alia, under the Beijing Declaration and the Platform for Action of the Fourth World Conference on Women, the Programme of Action of the International Conference on Population and Development and the Vienna Declaration and Programme of Action adopted by the World Conference on Human Rights;

(c) To collect and disseminate basic data about the occurrence of traditional or customary practices affecting the health of women and girls, including female genital mutilation;

(d) To develop, adopt and implement national legislation and policies that prohibit traditional or customary practices affecting the health of

women and girls, including female genital mutilation, and to prosecute the perpetrators of such practices;
(e) To establish or strengthen support services to respond to the needs of victims by, *inter alia*, developing comprehensive and accessible sexual and reproductive health services and providing training to healthcare providers at all levels on the harmful health consequences of such practices;
(f) To establish, if they have not done so, a concrete national mechanism for the implementation and monitoring of relevant legislation, law enforcement and national policies;
(g) To intensify efforts to raise awareness of and to mobilise international and national public opinion concerning the harmful effects of traditional or customary practices affecting the health of women and girls, including female genital mutilation, in particular through education, the dissemination of information, training, the media, the arts and local community meetings, in order to achieve the total elimination of these practices;
(h) To promote the inclusion of the discussion of the empowerment of women and their human rights in primary and secondary education curricula and to address specifically traditional or customary practices affecting the health of women and girls in such curricula and in the training of health personnel;
(i) To promote men's understanding of their roles and responsibilities with regard to promoting the elimination of harmful practices, such as female genital mutilation;
(j) To involve, among others, public opinion leaders, educators, religious leaders, chiefs, traditional leaders, medical practitioners, women's health and family planning organisations, the arts and the media in publicity campaigns with a view to promoting a collective and individual awareness of the human rights of women and girls and of how harmful traditional or customary practices violate those rights;
(k) To continue to take specific measures to increase the capacity of communities, including immigrant and refugee communities, in which female genital mutilation is practiced, to engage in activities aimed at preventing and eliminating such practices;
(l) To explore, through consultations with communities and religious and cultural groups and their leaders, alternatives to harmful traditional or customary practices, in particular where those practices form part of a ritual ceremony or rite of passage;
(m) To cooperate closely with the Special Rapporteur of the Sub-commission on the Promotion and Protection of Human Rights on

traditional practices affecting the health of women and the girl child and to respond to her inquiries;
(n) To cooperate closely with relevant specialised agencies and United Nations funds and programmes, as well as with relevant non-governmental and community organisations, in a joint effort to eradicate traditional or customary practices affecting the health of women and girls;
(o) To include in their reports to CEDAW, the Committee on the Rights of the Child and other relevant treaty bodies specific information on measures taken to eliminate traditional or customary practices affecting the health of women and girls, including female genital mutilation, and to prosecute the perpetrators of such practices. (UN 2000, p. 4)

This is significant as member states are asked to adopt and implement policies presented by the UN to reduce harmful cultural practices.

UNFPA makes the link between women, human rights and AIDS on its website:

> Violence against women has been called the most pervasive yet least recognised human rights abuse in the world. The Vienna Human Rights Conference and the Fourth World Conference on Women also gave priority to this issue and Violence against women is both a cause and consequence of AIDS. Research has confirmed a strong correlation between sexual and other forms of abuse against women and women's chances of contracting HIV. Male (or female) condoms are irrelevant when a woman is being beaten and raped. Moreover, forced vaginal penetration increases the likelihood of HIV transmission. In addition, the fear of violence prevents many women from asking their partners to use condoms, accessing HIV information, and from getting tested and seeking treatment, even when they strongly suspect they have been infected. Many women are in danger of being beaten, abandoned or thrown out of their homes if the HIV-positive status is known. If HIV-prevention activities are to succeed, they need to occur alongside other efforts that address and reduce violence against women and girls. (UNFPA 2013)

In 2000, a conference report produced by the United Nations' Educational, Scientific and Cultural Organisation (UNESCO), identified a number of key 'cultural features' of relevance in HIV prevention, treatment and care in Central and Southern Africa. These were identified as:

Individual-Based (premarital sex, extra marital sex, infertility, forced sex, sex for pleasure, life skills, fatalism, poverty, unemployment and migration); Family-Based (extended families, forced marriages, widow inheritance, domestic violence, gender relations, female genital mutilation and unemployment); Community Based (complacency, discrimination, fears and stigma, social exclusion, traditional healers and medicine, perception and interpretation of illness, illiteracy, poverty, herbal medicine, crime, alcohol and substance abuse); and Institutional Cooperation—Religious institutions and leadership, cultural leaders, NGOs and decentralisation. The report states:

> These country assessments have revealed important advancements in the use of the cultural approach to health development. The Conference has noted that cultural factors can be used to mitigate the impact of HIV/AIDS, if effectively integrated policies and programmes are focused at individual, family, community and at national/international levels. Pilot and case studies have shown that interventions at these levels can make significant improvement in the fight against HIV/AIDS. (UNESCO 2001, p. 7)

The paragraphs above demonstrate how global policies address issues of gender-based violence, harmful cultural practices and AIDS and how the UN has called upon member states to adopt measures to address them. What is confusing and blurred in these policy documents is exactly how the links are or are not understood between Harmful Cultural Practices, Gender-Based Violence and AIDS. The documents often (as shown above) claim these practices are detrimental to gender equality and breach human rights. Confusingly, many declarations and resolutions exist that focus on 'gender-based violence', 'harmful cultural practices' and 'HIV/AIDS', without clearly articulating the link between them. This is unhelpful for national governments that are expected to implement these policies.

How Did Malawi Respond to Global Policies?

At the 63rd UN General Assembly session in 2008 agenda item 56 was on the Advancement of Women. Under this heading the committee discussed: (i) Trafficking in women and girls; (ii) Intensification of efforts to eliminate all forms of violence against women; (iii) Eliminating rape and other forms of sexual violence in all their manifestations, including in conflict and related situation; and (iv) Improvement of the status of women in the United Nations system. In Malawi's statement to the UN on this agenda item, gender-based violence was highlighted as a problem for women and girls in Malawi, which, according to the statement, reinforces the subordination of women and promotes sexual abuse which leads to injury, HIV infection and unwanted pregnancies. The statement also highlighted one of the challenges Malawi faced as it is:

> weighed down by gaps between commitment and implementation coupled with continuing contradictions between customary laws, national laws and international commitments. (United Nations Malawi 2008, p. 2)

This section shows that at the international level, policies are explicitly identifying harmful cultural practices as an obstacle to women's empowerment and reducing women's vulnerability to AIDS. It has also shown how, pressure from international frameworks to deliver policies is juxtaposed with the national political landscape in Malawi in which, as this chapter highlights, national laws seem to reflect the elitist views of a few. International policies differ to implementation at the national level revealing differences in the way actors at these levels perceive the AIDS and harmful cultural practices narrative. At the national level complex internal hierarchies are at play out of which flow rather distorted narratives on who is to blame and why for Malawi's high prevalence of HIV. I will now look at policies on harmful cultural practices, AIDS and gender-based violence in Malawi highlighting this disjuncture between how they are talked about in global documents and national frameworks.

National Policies on Harmful Cultural Practices and AIDS in Malawi

In this section I show that the Government of Malawi oversimplifies links between AIDS, violence and harmful cultural practices. I also show how the Government drafted new legislation on AIDS to eradicate harmful cultural practices because of the imagined link between harmful cultural practices and AIDS. The legislation emerged as a response to pressure from international donors as shown above.

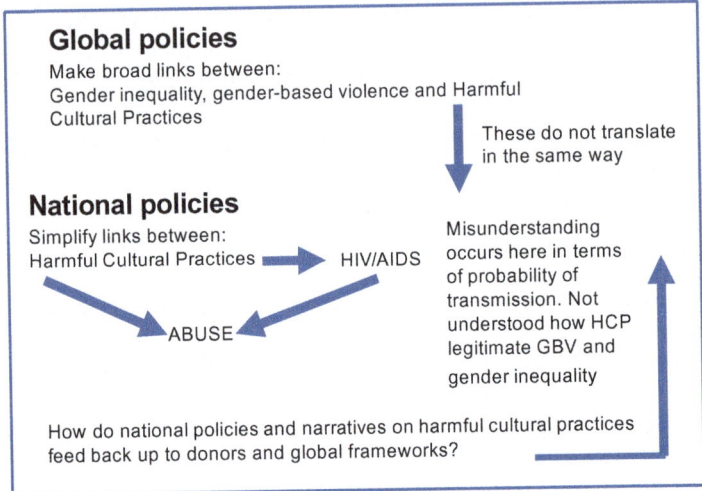

Fig. 4.1 Difference between global policies on gender-based violence, harmful cultural practices and AIDS and those at the national level (*Source* Author)

In Malawi's national HIV policy. It states that:

> Some customary practices increase the risk of HIV infection. Among these are polygamy, extramarital sexual relations, marital rape, first aid to snake-bite victims, ear piercing and tattooing (mphini), and traditional practices such as widow- and widower- inheritance (*chokolo*), death cleansing (*kupita kufa*), forced sex for young girls coming of age (*fisi*), newborn cleansing (*kutenga mwana*), circumcision (*jando* or *mdulidwe*), ablution of dead bodies, consensual adultery for childless couples (*fisi*), wife and husband exchange (*chimwanamaye*) and temporary husband replacement (*mbulo*). (GoM 2003, p. 21)

In Fig. 4.1 I show that at the national level a direct link is made between sexual cultural practices and increased risk of HIV infection. This is different from the UN's interpretation. At the international level, we saw earlier with the UN political declaration on HIV/AIDS that the links are not articulated so clearly and where the concern is not so much that practices directly lead to sharp increases in HIV rates, but that they sustain an environment in which women are vulnerable to violence. Sexual violence is known to lead to higher transmission rates—not the practices themselves.

The following statement highlights the direct link the Malawian government made about harmful cultural practices and AIDS:

> Government, through the NAC, undertakes to do the following:
>
> - in partnership with civil society including religious leaders, sensitise traditional leaders and their subjects on the dangers of customary practices such as death cleansing (kupita kufa), forced sex for young girls coming of age (fisi or kuchotsa fumbi), newborn cleansing (kutenga mwana), consensual adultery for childless couples (fisi), wife- and husband-exchange (chimwanamaye), temporary husband replacement (mbulo), and sucking of blood (to help snakebite victims), all of which practices may lead to HIV infection.
> - ensure that traditional leaders stop or modify unsafe customary practices to make them safer in order to prevent HIV transmission, or promote alternative customary practices which do not place people at risk of HIV infection. (GoM 2003, p. 21)

In 2006 a special Law Commission was set up in Malawi to develop a new piece of legislation on AIDS. In 2008 a report entitled 'Report of the Law Commission on the Development of HIV/AIDS Legislation' was published. In this report it states:

> At the UN General Assembly in June, 2001, Heads of Governments agreed that strong leadership at all levels of society is essential for an effective response to the epidemic: leadership by Governments in combatting HIV/AIDS is essential and their efforts should be complemented by the full and active participation of civil society, the business community and the private sector; and that leadership involves personal commitment and concrete actions. Following these recommendations of UN General Assembly, the NACP [National AIDS Control Programme] was replaced by a new institution, the National AIDS Commission (NAC) in July, 2001, which was constituted as a public trust. (Malawi Law Commission 2008, p. 8)

This demonstrates that as a result of the UN General Assembly Special Session on AIDS in 2001, the Government of Malawi decided to make a fundamental shift in the way that AIDS was being addressed in the country, establishing the NAC to report directly to the Office of the President and Cabinet. This was done with 'a view to bringing the highest political office to commit fully to fighting the epidemic and to ensure Government oversight activities at the highest political level' (Malawi Law Commission 2008, p. 8).

According to the report, the basis for HIV reform was a result of two submissions made to the Law Commission: one from the Department of Nutrition and HIV/AIDS calling for a legislative framework to govern AIDS issues and one from the NAC calling for a legislative institutional framework to allow it to function. The special Commission was established for several reasons including developing a new piece of legislation on AIDS. The report explains why:

> The Commission opted to develop a new piece of legislation on HIV/AIDS principally because the Commission considered the issue of HIV/AIDS as a cross-cutting multi-sectoral issue and as such inappropriate to be tackled under the existing piece of legislation. Secondly, the Commission considered that the proposed law on HIV/AIDS combine issues of prevention and management of HIV/AIDS. (Malawi Law Commission 2008, p. 9)

This is an important point as the Commission refers to HIV/AIDS prevention. However, perhaps as a result of global development policies and the call by the UN for member states 'to develop, adopt and implement national legislation and policies that prohibit traditional or customary practices affecting the health of women and girls' (2000, p. 2, see also, p. 77), influenced the Government of Malaw's decision to draft a new piece of legislation on AIDS to change specific cultural practices.

I interviewed a lawyer from the Law Commission who holds a Master's degree. He told me:

> This reform has come about as a result of various international fora including Cairo ICPD 1994 and Beijing Platform for Action, 1995. It is also stated in the Constitution under Chapter IV human rights Sections 20 and 24. In 1994 a new constitution was introduced including a Bill of Rights. This was a period of new thinking in which human rights needed to be unpacked. (P23)

When I attended a Parliamentary Committee Meeting on AIDS that was considering the proposed legislation, a Lawyer from the Malawi Law Commission stated that the UN raised issues of criminalisation that he thought were pertinent and should be included in the legislation. The Chair proposed that the points made from the floor were taken into consideration and included in the proposed legislation at the Secretariat. The MPs agreed. (Journal entry, 13 January 2009)

The report states:

> The vulnerability of women and girls to HIV/AIDS is aggravated by certain cultural and religious practices. The Commission further observed that such practices not only violate the dignity of females but are usually practiced without the express consent of women and befall females mainly on the basis of their sex or marital status. The Commission observed that while the rights to participate in a culture of choice is protected under the Constitution, in most cases, women participate in cultural practices without given fee consent due to high dependency on men as wives, mistresses and children. The Commission noted that beyond exacerbating the spread of HIV/AIDS, these harmful practices violate women's rights and also denigrate as such. To this end the Commission concluded that these practices were discriminatory against women. (Malawi Law Commission 2008, p. 33)

The customs and practices in question include widow inheritance, widow cleansing, sexual relations associated with initiation or rites of passage and swapping of spouses, among others. Most of the cultural practices involve sex.

The Commission noted the State's obligation to introduce legislation, in particular relating to culture, for the purpose of guaranteeing the exercise and enjoyment of human rights and fundamental freedoms on the basis of equality of the women (see article 3 of the CEDAW). The Protocol also urges State parties to prohibit and condemn all forms of harmful practices which negatively affect the rights of women and which are contrary to recognised human rights standards (Article 5 CEDAW). With respect to sexual and reproductive rights, the Protocol urges State parties to observe a number of rights of women in connection with AIDS including the right to self protection and protection from sexually transmitted infection including AIDS: and the right to be informed of the health status of her partner, particularly if he is infected with AIDS Article 14(1). The Commission observed that during consultations participants were generally in agreement with the prohibition of practices that are perceived to spread HIV infection. Participants, however, were divided on the issue of polygamy (p. 34).

Section 24 of the Constitution required the State to pass legislation to eliminate customs and practices that discriminate against women and this legislation was passed in 2010. The National AIDS Policy outlaws customs and practices that perpetuate the risk of infection with HIV. The Commission recommended that any person who subjects another person to a harmful cultural practice shall be guilty of an offence and liable to a fine of 100,000 Malawian Kwacha and imprisonment for five years. Under the 'First Schedule' 18 so-called harmful practices are listed. These are: 1. Chimwanamaye (wife and husband swapping), 2. Fisi (forced sex for young girls coming of age; consensual adultery for childless couples), 3. Hlazi (bonus wife), 4. **Chijura mphinga**,[1] 5. Kuchotsa fumbi (a girl having sex with a boy to 'remove the dust' (MHRC), 6. Chiharo (wife inheritance), 7. Kuika mwana Kumalo (when a girl falls pregnant she is asked to sleep with a man in order for the child to grow well), 8. Kujura nthowa (to open the way), 9. Kulowa kufa (a man sleeps with a woman whose husband or son had just died, to put to rest the spirit of the deceased) (MHRC), 10. **Kulowa ku ngozi**, 11. Kupimbira (young girls are given in marriage to wealthy old men as payment for their parents' debts or for other purposes—MHRC), 12. Kupondera guwa, 13. Kusamala mlendo, 14. **Kutsuka mwana**, 15. Mbirigha (bonus wife) (MHRC), 16. Gwamula (young men invade kuka (girls' dormitory) at night and force the girls to have sex with them) (MHRC), 17. Bulganeti la mfumu (pimping of a young virgin to a visiting traditional leader), 18. **Mwana akule**.[2]

The lawyer (P23) carried out most of the preparatory work for two pieces of proposed legislation; one on gender equality and one on AIDS. He told me that the pieces of legislation differ as follows: (1) gender equality is related to harm with respect to women in terms of women based purely on their sex. This may include STIs. (2) HIV/AIDS is related to harm with respect to HIV infection.

Cultural practices, he said, have to be covered under both laws. The idea is not to have a case by case study but that the issue of cultural practices falls 'within realm of social regulation'. I asked about evidence to inform decisions to implement the two laws. He said it is not an issue of evidence-based research but rather 'an issue of risk'. This is interesting given my emphasis on the lack of evidence. He clearly says it's not necessary. We talked about the probability of transmission of HIV. 'The truth is in our Commission they told us that it is not very likely from one sexual act'. He said that 'statistics are figures that may just apply to you'. In other words if there is one per cent chance of contracting the disease then you may be the one per cent. He pointed out that the issue is also about age of sexual debut. 'Therefore infants may not take levels of precaution'. As a result there is an 'exposure element' which is taken into account rather than the actual risk. In other words children have the right to be protected from all risk—however high or low (P23).

We talked about different types of '*fisi*'—Initiation '*fisi*' and conception '*fisi*'. He said for the initiation '*fisi*' prohibition and regulation both come into play. 'If you are caught then you are punished'. I asked what is the punishment? 'Punishment is imprisonment but if the *fisi* is HIV+ then the punishment is more severe.' I asked about the Commission to which he referred. It was set up in 2007. It comprised an academic who is 'a PLWHA'; a Pathologist; a Priest; a retired civil servant; a representative from NAPHAM; the Head of NAC; a Minister, a representative from Ministry of Justice, a Law Commissioner and two lawyers from the Law Commission. He described it as 'an ad hoc group that has now disbanded'. Members' selection was based on 'relevance and expertise and involvement in the subject' (P23).

I then asked which type of law do 'cultural practices' fall under? This appeared to be a contentious issue. Some agreed and some disagreed that it falls under criminal law. In terms of developing the proposed legislation the Commission adopted three approaches: not to ignore criminal law approach; look at human rights approach and address public health law. There is a law on public health, which was introduced in 1948, that does not include AIDS. The public health law does deal with all curable diseases which he described as 'explosive diseases' i.e. tuberculosis, cholera. He said that HIV is different – 'the manifestation of the disease is different' (P23). He said a largely accepted hypothesis by the Parliamentary Committee is that a 'fusion' between public health and criminal law is needed (P23). Here we see how AIDS has been treated as an exceptional disease, to which I have referred in Chapter 3.

He explained there are turbulent times in Parliament regarding passing of laws and big problems as during the last five years not many bills have been passed. I asked where the idea came from to implement such reforms. The idea for the new legislation came from the gender-related laws reform programme, which originally came from the Law

Commission. There are three parts to this programme: 1. Inheritance and succession, 2. Report of the law commission on the review of the laws on marriage and divorce, and 3. Gender equality.

The Law Commission drafts reports, which are then presented to government. They are 'gazetted'—an endorsement process by government which means they are now a public record. The Cabinet then looks at the document and makes a decision. The document is then presented to Parliament as a government bill, and given a first reading then a second reading. It then goes to the legislature because it has been adopted by government, and an arm of legislation then enacts it. I asked when does he expect the legislation on cultural practices will be passed. He said he thought it may happen after the elections in May 2009 (the law was passed in 2010). At the time there were many bills waiting to be passed. For example, the Criminal Law Bill had been waiting to be passed since 1998. The lawyer went on to provide his critique of the bills. He made two points. First, he said Malawi is not a heavily regulated country. There is a certain freedom to do what one wants beyond the law. He says even if a law is passed it does not mean it is enacted upon but 'looks good in statute books'. Second, he added that there is a strong donor influence to 'do this and do that' and that is why certain pieces of legislation are being drafted (P23). This is an important point as it demonstrates the key role donors play in influencing national policy. Further, whereas there is evidence that there is a process of policy scrutiny there seems very little evidence that such a process has any tangible outcomes on changing policy.

He talked about issues of regulating HIV testing and counselling. He mentioned a discussion concerning a law to introduce compulsory testing for pregnant women. He said the 'NGOs were up in arms'. He talked about another donor approach, couple testing—that women need to get tested with their husbands. But he said what is really happening is that women are 'hiring spouses' to attend the clinic with them. However, it is totally implausible that these men, even if they came to the clinic, would be tested. This probably reflects the practice of families hiring *fisi*.

He said there are positive aspects of cultural values but there seems to be 'a quest to destroying everything'. He is not specific about who is doing the destroying but given the context of the conversation he seems to be applying responsibility to donors. He continued by explaining that 'There is also a pressure to modernise and things are moving faster than society is. If you kill a practice you erase a value and create a vacuum which is difficult to fill'. He said 'What is the principle behind it? How does it affect everyone else?' He felt the country should bring in regulation rather than prohibition. He talked about law reform and what law reform actually means. He described it as 'urban legislation – legislation for the elite'.

He started to explain *Chokolo*. He said that *Chokolo* is defined as the person who is inherited whereas *Chiharo* is the actual practice. He gave an example of a brother's death. If his brother dies he is responsible for the wife. Some men choose to have sex with the wife which is 'chauvinistic'. However, not all men do and the man may just provide financial support. So if *Chokolo* is prohibited the wife stops receiving support. He said there is a need to be open-minded.

He told me he attended a meeting in Blantyre, which was trying to 'sensitise' chiefs on cultural practices. During the meeting the chiefs said that they have changed the cultural practices. Then while he was having a one-to-one with a chief, the chief whispered in his ear 'Why are you trying to take away our privileges?' Privileges here could mean that men have carte blanche to have sex with young girls or women who have started their first menses. The chief is referring to taking away their privileges by not allowing them to have sex with young women. Another person interviewed said: 'But also the traditional leaders themselves, although they might hide information, sometimes they can slip off the tongue and tell you some stuff' (P25). Traditional leaders may not be telling the truth but instead telling those who visit the villages what they think they want to hear, e.g., that the practice is no longer carried out.

One problem with the piece of legislation is how to monitor it as implementation and monitoring is difficult given the secrecy surrounding sexual cultural practices.

P5 Interview with a Member of Parliament, PhD

Aaah I was there for a long time and even when we had our own way of coordinating our activities on HIV/AIDS, we were forced to abandon that and take the approved structure by the World Bank and create the National Aids Commission in the way it is now. Aaa, soo, international NGOs have played a big role in fact they call it policy dialogue but it was not really a dialogue but it was a monologue aah so, that's one.

I think aaah, eeeh there has been a lot of international pressure on what the programme on HIV/AIDS should be, aaa, there is also much concern about HIV/AIDS and money of course came from rich countries and big international organisations. And really the agenda was dictated by the international world.

Yaah, when we started the fight against HIV/AIDS the most difficult community that I met were the religious community, the faith-based community later on that's how it was labelled. I conducted a workshop for them, in 2000 I think, February, I was lucky because then I was vice president so I could add some power to command (laughter). And I chaired it myself. I said I wanted bishops, the highest echelon of Christianity as well and the Islamic organisations and they responded. We were in the Capital Hotel for eleven hours, I said nobody is going out; no one is going out, if you wanted tea it would be brought in and in that room toilets are inside there, so you just go at the back (laughter). So it was tough, but at the end we, we had an agenda at the end we had twelve points that we said we should discuss I don't remember all of them but they thought I was making it wrong, of course one point about condoms which could, and therefore, Catholic bishops could not … but we agreed that you know, alright, this on the pulpit, we are not saying that you go and talk about condoms but also respect our responsibility as government to inform the population so don't preach against us. (P5)

The passage above P5 says that international NGOs influenced the policy process and that the World Bank exerted pressure to create a NAC. The statement from this respondent fits within my argument concerning donor influence on the policy process (see Chapter 3 where I provide a critique of the World Bank and Structural Adjustment Policies and aid conditionality). For example the MP describes how the Government of Malawi was forced to abandon their own plans and replace them with a structure approved by the World Bank. What would have been interesting to know is what would have happened if the Government of Malawi had decided to continue with their own plans. Would funding have been withdrawn by the World Bank? Because the World Bank injects significant funds in Malawi in the prevention of HIV and AIDS, the Government of Malawi may have been careful not to offend or challenge the donor. Furthermore, because the Government of Malawi lacks financial power it may only play a limited role in policymaking. This passage also throws doubts on the assumption in policy analysis that national governments are completely in control of their public policymaking processes.

A respondent working for ActionAid who has a Bachelor of Arts degree made several important points (see P36 interview with a Policy Advisor): women not knowing that a law exists because they are illiterate; problems with accessing information as well as dealing with the judicial processes and the perpetrators. She highlights that even if policies were implemented to protect women from violence, the women may be unaware of the laws that are there to protect them. She also highlights the difficulty for women to proceed with court cases as she says those making decisions are men and these men will protect other men and not listen to women and see their issues as 'gender nonsense'.

P36 Interview with a Policy Advisor

Because a piece of legislation doesn't do anything if you don't report it, and if I don't know about it, it doesn't do anything. So there is that gap, that major challenge in terms of implementing and most[3] of the people that we deal with they are illiterate, they can't read. So that's one challenge in terms of the gap. Filling the gap between the policies that are there and the grassroots that cannot read. And the other challenge is women's actual participation, actual participation in terms of women knowing that these laws are there to protect them. And sometimes you find that ya, we don't have a lot of justice delivery mechanism ya, where you should walk ten kilometres to access justice. I mean, it becomes a challenge because if I'm raped, it means it's already a problem and for me to walk ten kilometres to and fro and it's a frustrating process because you are told come back! come back! Come back, you know, the following day. So people give up easily. So we don't have local Justice delivery systems that are effective. And you find that the chiefs are mostly men, men who would want to protect their fellow citizens..., men –who have perpetrated aah... So there is that challenge in terms of getting the chief's buy in to protect women. To use the law to protect women. To understand the laws but also to protect women to be pro-women because some of them they don't listen they just no! this is gender nonsense. You know they... they... they switch off. Ya. And then the other challenge in terms of, the police. The police they don't have capacity especially for the case. You find that when you report a case it takes very long for you to get to the court. So it's not like instant. And sometimes you get threats from the person who has perpetrated you and there is no protection. The protection is not forthcoming so you are afraid you withdraw the case or you know you get tired. You get frustrated in the long run. So there is that I don't know what you can call it. That disconnect in terms of what the law can say, can provide in terms of provision and what really happens on the ground. (P36)

The P25 interview with a Programme Officer, UNAIDS, illustrates the challenges governments face to implement policy at the national level. She says that the Ministry of Women wanted a piece of legislation drafted on cultural practices but as she highlights it would be difficult to implement it because of the traditional leaders' forum. This highlights the challenges governments face working with national groups, in this case the traditional leaders' forum, who exert a considerable amount of power.

> Having legislation is one thing but we are grappling with the actual translating of these laws into practice and actually being able to apply them. Usually when they are drafting these laws they have a special commission which is supposed to consult whatever; so I think there might be a group of people who are already doing that, I haven't been consulted. Even in the Ministry of Women I think they wanted to have as a piece of legislation on cultural issues. Maybe they had to do something - the ministry, because of too many of the cultural practices that, I mean I am talking from the perspective that I find. It's a good idea but somewhere let's look at how best we are implementing the legislations that are in place right now, you know, then go further if we see that there is no other way because otherwise the traditional leaders forum it's like we are killing ourselves in the foot as well, you know, because we think we're hoping that this group can be of influence on a lot of communities because they have a lot of power. But can we come with the legislation unit, yes, now saying ok the state is saying this but if you do it, it will go further down because the leaders feel like they are left out, you know. So, they can be able to address cultural issues without really having to go, unless they are completely, probably out of context, you know, they are really not doing anything. (P25)

A lawyer told me about her own research on polygamy:

> When you look at the sort of statistics I found, you find that in some cases polygamy was highly practiced in areas where they had said it is illegal. Whereas in the countries where they had said it is legal, in some cases you saw that the percentages of polygamy were low. So I say to myself, what could be the ratio. And I also made an analogy, which is not in my thesis, with female genital mutilation; in some areas they tried to go the legislative way and ban it, but to find that the prevalence rate of female genital mutilation was actually higher than in the areas where they had said ok, let's not legislate against it. Now, the law commission will tell you 'what was the missing point?'; the missing point is, and this is what we say the

law commission, you cannot really successfully legislate on culture, practices that are embedded on culture unless you adopt a very comprehensive or holistic approach, whereby that kind of legislation should be complemented by other non-legislative measures. I am sure you have already looked at this kind of issue in your study, to say 'do we have an inspective civic education mode for this kind of practice?' civic education, empowerment, because, if we talk of civic education per say where at least the majority of the population you are targeting is educated then they will begin to appreciate the issues to say 'oh, probably this is why this kind of practice should be abandoned'. Civic educate them so that they begin to appreciate the issues, so that we don't just impose on them to say this is that, ought to stop it. Empower them because you most variably find that where these kinds of practices are highly practiced because people believe in some value that is attached to them. So, for example, polygamy, female genital mutilation, it's all a means of securing marriage, I need to stay in marriage; but if people are empowered economically and with information they begin to see that probably a marriage is not all there is, I can survive outside of a marriage, you know. So, I said in my thesis that we need a holistic approach which should complement the legislation element. Other than that, we just drive the practice underground and it is heavily practiced and it is risky and dangerous, because now that you've made it illegal, people will no longer come into the office and say you see they did this to me and it offers all room for all kinds of abuse. So, that's how I looked at it, and in our submission to the Malawi Law Commission we said as much.

Then the other issue is, we look at international human rights instrument, what have they said the CEDAW, the Protocol, to the African charter of women, you will see that the emphasis is on eliminating harmful cultural practices, in some instances modifying. I will emphasise harmful, you know, first you have to do the kind of research you are doing then you will conclude is this harmful. After that stage, you'll say what's the best way of handling the issue; elimination or modification. So for example, in Kenya, on the issue of female genital mutilation, they did a pilot study where they said 'should we eliminate female genital mutilation? Their answer was to look at the values that underpin the practice. And they found that it was actually an avenue where girls were given the necessary information as they get the rite of *passage to womanhood*. So they said, we cannot do away with this because it's actually a source of informal education, most of the girls in the rural areas do not go to school anyway; so if we find a grouping where we can put them together and give them the right information. They modified the practice in that they were to have the initiation ceremonies without the cutting but including HIV/AIDS messages into the information package, and it was actually improved now to say, the current issues in the society. So, at the end of the day, you had these girls who would go out into the public and say we've been initiated and be acceptable culturally, but without the harmful element. I am not sure if the Malawi Law commission did that kind of approach, to examine each and every cultural practice and to say this is harmful in this regard, let us recommend for its modification, or there is nothing we can do to this except for its elimination, I'm not sure if that was done; we made that kind of submission to them (they receive all sorts of submission, and what they do with them we really can't tell, you can only do so much). (P26)

In this section I have shown how international frameworks are difficult to implement on the ground and how the Government of Malawi has struggled to balance the expectations of the donors with their understanding of Malawian perspectives. Complex legislation emerges which has little resemblance to realities on ground and is certainly not supported by evidence. The legislation does however satisfy donors who are happy to see money channelled into programmes conceived to realise the laws.

The Malawian Elite

In this section I look at the role of the Malawian elite in constructing policy on AIDS and sexual cultural practices and how they position themselves in the development industry in relation to international donors. Literature in the international development field about national elites is difficult to find. There is not much on those who are the conduits of resources and information from the offices in the capital of international organisations such as World Bank, USAID, DFID, World Vision to their branch offices. Elites control the flow of information between INGOs and national government departments. The country nationals are crucial—the big donors cannot do anything without them, and alternatively the big donors rely on people in their national offices for information (e.g. what programmes are needed, what programmes that they implemented were successful what not) (Swidler and Watkins 2009). International donors develop policy and fund programmes based on very little information about what goes on in Malawi, which is a concern – this is the case even when the INGOs do have district-level offices.

Malawians who work in the development field can be described as elites (Watkins and Swidler 2009; Myroniuk 2011). They stand out from the average Malawian as educated to secondary and tertiary levels.

They are involved in the distribution and implementation of millions of pounds on aid; they are also those on whom international expectations fall to decrease the transmission of HIV (Myroniuk 2011). They are part of a small, relatively well-off economic and social strata. The response to the AIDS epidemic in Malawi was a flood of NGOs (Morfit 2011). These NGOs required educated staff: thus, funding from international donors that passed through NGOs substantially increased the opportunities for jobs in the AIDS sector. In order to qualify for a position one must be able to speak English and be literate. The research of Swidler and Watkins (2017) categories the elites into three groups: national elites who staff NGOs in the capital, district elites who are engaged in implementing NGO projects in the districts, and interstitial elites who have secondary school but have difficulty finding a job with a stable salary.

This next section describes how the national and district elites maintain jobs and their status by framing narratives of the causes of the AIDS epidemic. The jobs of the civil servants are secure, but the jobs in the NGOs are not: an NGO may be closed because the NGO has no more funding, or they may vanish because of corruption.

In an interview with a national elite at the NAC, I asked him what his job entails. He said, 'Facilitating partnerships, mainstreaming, capacity building'. I asked what does this actually mean? He said it means 'Providing guidance, development of policies and strategies on those areas and providing technical assistance in those areas and monitoring how effective those are' (P35). This interview illustrated the pivotal role of elites as they act to transform donor policies and to turn these policies into programmes on the ground.

I interviewed a Communications Officer working for GOAL based in Blantyre. He has a Bachelor of Arts Degree. He was born in the city because his father used to work for a company that involved moving from one place to another so time and again they made a point to see people, his grandparents. When I asked "where did you go to secondary school?" He said: 'I think it was just natural but uh since from standard 1 you don't have a choice your parents say go to school so we get to standard 8 and then you proceed to secondary school'. What is striking about his response is he says it was just natural. He is telling me that he is elite as he took it for granted that he would go to secondary school. He then tells me:

> Since graduation I have worked for two organisations the first one was Malawi Writers Union. It was an arts and culture organisation. I worked as a Project Officer. Later on I was editor for an arts and culture magazine which they introduced while I was still there. I worked there for two years. Afterwards then I joined GOAL. (P1)

When I asked him about his job, I hear development jargon—'cross cutting, middle managers, communication mechanisms'.

P34 Partnership and Liaison Officer

P34 has worked at NAC for five years. Prior to NAC he worked for Plan International as a Programme Coordinator on livelihoods and HIV/AIDS. He was also a local United Nations Volunteer (UNV) at UNDP. He said he 'got paid handsomely' doing emergency fieldwork – he then corrected himself to say 'more correct to say 'humanitarian affairs'. He worked at UNDP for one and a half years based in Nkhata Bay. The UNV contract was for two years; the maximum time one can be a volunteer. But he left early to 'follow his wife' as she had a permanent job. He said his time at UNDP was 'enriching'. Malawi at the time was experiencing a hunger crisis. He said 'I was at the forefront providing situational analysis for whole country'. He holds a Bachelor's degree. After UNDP he worked for USAID as a regional coordinator in Lilongwe working on electoral monitoring -this was five years ago. He was working on the electoral support system and remained in the post for six months only. When I asked him why he only worked for six months he said the contract was only for nine months so he left to find another job. He also worked for Plan International and UNDP in related fields. I asked him why the NAC. He said two things. One because of the area of focus – HIV/AIDS. He said UNDP was a 'vulnerable continuation'. He also said that the perks at NAC are higher than USAID and the contract longer – three years. He said the salary is higher and that it is possible to renew contract after three years. He said he wants to stay at NAC. He added that the organisation has to be interested in keeping you as well.

In both these cases two issues are apparent. The high demand these elites are in from international stakeholders and the short-term nature of their work. These same two factors characterise the career of my next respondent.

Case Study of a Programme Officer

Education and career of a Programme Officer working for GOAL Malawi

P7 and his colleague greeted me at the bus depot in Balaka. The office was closed as it was Christmas holidays but he was happy to meet me on his day off. We made our way to a motel to hold the interview. P3 from GOAL Blantyre suggested I meet with P7.

P7's father is from Zomba and his mother is from Machinga but both parents are now in Machinga. He attended secondary school and then got a degree in nursing. He worked at a private hospital for two years, then moved to take a position at an NGO where he was involved in and HIV/AIDS project and HIV/AIDS activities like Prevention of Mother To Child Transmission (PMTCT), home-based care and then he was responsible for an Infection Prevention Programme, and he was heading that department at a district hospital. He said he was with the NGO working "hand in hand" with the hospital trying to support them. He was also responsible for the ARV programme.

After close to three years the programme (the mission) which they were running came to an end. The Mission was closed so he moved to GOAL Malawi to work on an HIV/AIDS programme. Initially he was responsible for PMTCT, HIV Testing and Counselling and Home-Based Care for a district in southern Malawi. When asked how he felt about the programme coming to an end he said he had a good experience, he was exposed to many activities as far as HIV/AIDS programme is concerned but then at the end he heard that the mission was being closed when the project came to an end. It was a shock to him as he asked himself 'what am I going to do?' I need to find another job, I need to move out of this place, I have to go somewhere. I don't know what it will be like so finding a new job—it wasn't a nice experience.

I asked a staff member at NAC in terms of Behaviour Change Interventions do you think NAC is having an impact? He said, "It is probably best to talk to the people in Behaviour Change Interventions but so far so good as there are high levels of awareness about behaviour for example faithfulness". He also said that cultural dimensions underpin behaviour and that what we do is rooted in cultural beliefs. I asked him what he meant by cultural beliefs. He said, "There are so many in Malawi. Originally farmers had very good intentions – mostly to focus on the family but those norms and beliefs had to be redefined due to HIV. Because of levels of education especially in rural settings it is difficult to change cultural beliefs. The main problem of cultural beliefs is education, which form part and parcel of life. In urban areas they have changed them but if you go to villages they still exist and he said that the reason for that is because of levels of education". I asked him how he knows that. He said, "It is difficult to see and to interact with people. They say these are people from NAC let us tell them what they want to hear". A woman from Nsanje said 'these men are lying. Once these visitors go back, we will continue those practices' (P19). By blaming the uneducated villagers he is placing himself apart as a member of the urban and educated elite. The explanations provided by the elite not only help them secure longer contracts by ensuring donors fund more long-term programmes but also maintain the social hierarchy that keeps them in positions of decision-making power.

Narratives of Blame Among the Malawian Elite: 'Harmful Cultural Practices Spreading AIDS'

In this section I analyse interviews, training manuals and policy documents to evidence how the links between AIDS and harmful cultural practices are understood by the Malawian elite. Several pertinent issues are addressed in this section: how the 'Malawian elite', how they (the Malawian elite) perceive rural communities as backwards; the way the elites distance themselves from the villagers therefore demonstrating their 'eliteness'; their backwardness is given as the reason for cultural practices and are in turn blamed for the spread of HIV; this as argued previously is a distortion of reality.

I conducted an interview with a Cabinet Minister, who explained:

> There are initiation ceremonies that take place; the ceremonies like hyena. When somebody reaches puberty they initiate sexual intercourse. In relation to the cultural practices you find that young girls have their sexual debut at a very tender age. And that in many cases the new infections are higher in young girls. And it is because most of them are having the sexual intercourse with older men who may have already been infected so that is the *direct link between that and this one*.....Now when you look at that to be very honest with you in terms of policy, we are a little bit lagging behind. Because you do not expect a person like me to go out and deal

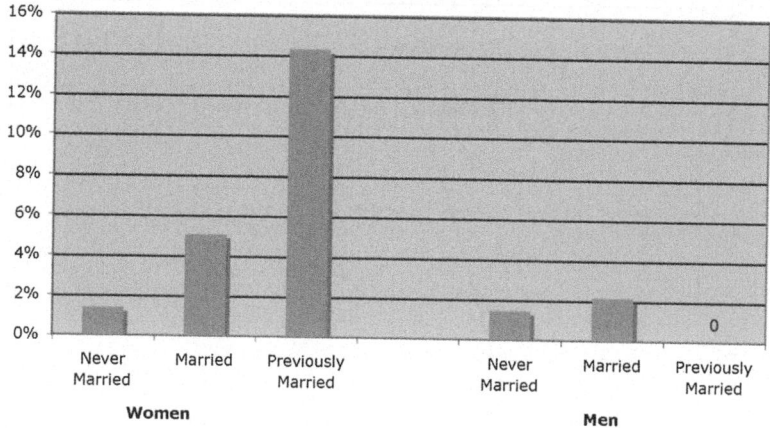

Fig. 4.2 HIV prevalence by gender and marital status (% HIV-Positive) among respondents aged 15–24, Malawi (*Source* Watkins [2010] based on data from the Malawi Diffusion and Ideational Change Project [MDICP 2004])

with those things. You need the traditional leaders like the chiefs, the traditional initiators, the traditional counsellors to deal with the problem. Let them understand it is an issue, let them understand that it is contributing to the spread of the disease of the HIV virus. (P41)

There are many inaccuracies in this passage; firstly, and as shown previously, while the incidence of new infections among people 15–24 is indeed higher among women than men in that age group, incidence among married women in that age groups is substantially higher. On the contrary, infections are higher among married and previously married women and there is now considerable evidence, both from Malawi and elsewhere in Sub-Saharan Africa, that marriage is a major risk factor for HIV—see Fig. 4.2 (UNAIDS 2004; MDHS 2010; Mkandawire-Valhmu et al. 2013).

A survey carried out by the MDICP at the University of Pennsylvania found that among respondents age 15–45, in three rural districts the prevalence rate for unmarried women was 1.5% while for married women it was 6.1% (MDICP, 2004). The probable explanation for lower HIV prevalence rates among unmarried women is that sex is infrequent; thus, given the low probability of transmission in a single act of intercourse, she is relatively unlikely to become infected.

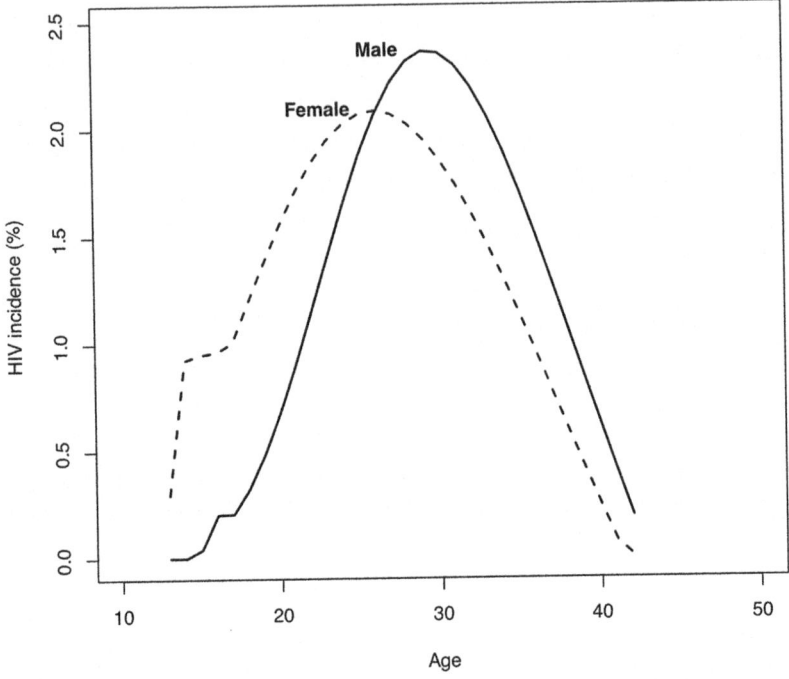

Fig. 4.3 HIV incidence by gender and age, all ages above age 15, Rural and Urban Malawi, demographic and health survey data, 2005 (*Source* Cited in Watkins [2010] Prepared by Patrick Gerland, United Nations Population Division, from DHS survey data)

Figure 4.3 shows incidence: what is highlighted from this figure is the importance of looking beyond ages 15–24. As demonstrated, women in Malawi appear to be more vulnerable to HIV when younger compared to men at older ages. This is probably due to men providing money or gifts that cost money, such as food and clothing, to wives, girls, sex workers, who are more likely to be HIV positive (Watkins 2010, p. 151).

Watkins made a comparative analysis of sex ratios of prevalence and incidence in other countries in sub-Saharan Africa where prevalence is high. She concluded that the basic transmission probability of HIV in a single act of intercourse varies little across countries. Her study compared Zambia and Tanzania, both countries bordering Malawi.

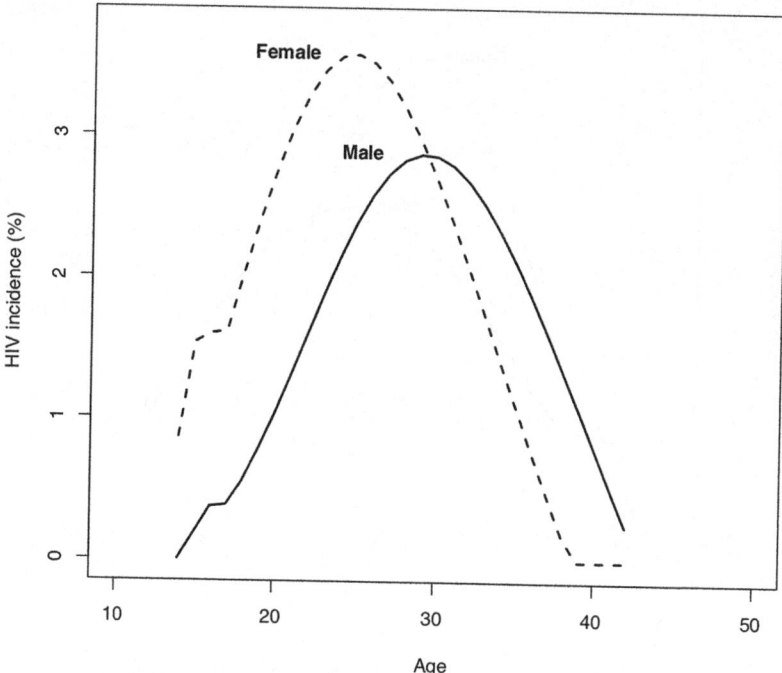

Fig. 4.4 HIV incidence by gender and age, all ages above age 15, Rural and Urban, Zambia, demographic and health survey data, 2001–2002 (*Source* Cited in Watkins [2010] Prepared by Patrick Gerland, United Nations Population Division, from DHS survey data)

She illustrates how Zambia and Tanzania are similar to Malawi in that there is a crossover in incidence, an age after which men are more likely to become infected than women—Figs. 4.4 and 4.5 (2010, p. 152).

A Cabinet Minister, P41, said most initiates are having sexual intercourse with older men who may have already been infected. The Minister, however, is incorrect. Although young Muslim male initiates are expected to have sex following the initiation period—which includes male circumcision—they are expected to have sex with Muslim girls in their own age group.

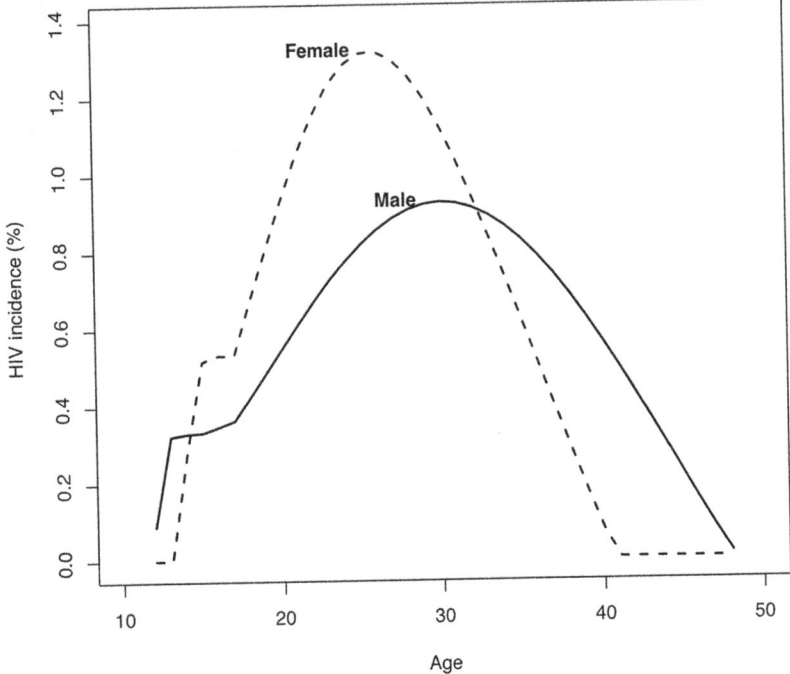

Fig. 4.5 HIV incidence by gender and age, all ages above age 15, Rural and Urban, Tanzania, demographic and health survey data, 2004–2005 (*Source* Cited in Watkins [2010] Prepared by Patrick Gerland, United Nations Population Division, from DHS survey data)

Interestingly the Cabinet Minister goes on to talk about policy, that Malawi is 'lagging behind' and that a person like her is not expected to deal with 'those things'. Rather, she puts responsibility of curbing the *fisi* practice back to the village chiefs to deal with the problem, that they should understand that the practice is contributing to the spread of HIV. I pointed out to the Minister that the NAC has policies in place to address HIV prevention and cultural practices. I said that I did not think anyone knew the extent to which the practice takes place in the country. She responded:

We have scanty information. That is why as an office we are saying we want a comprehensive nationwide study. So that because each district is unique in terms of cultural practices in its own way so we want to deal with them within that uniqueness. You can't say one jacket fits all the districts because of the background, the practices, the behaviours, they are totally different. (P41)

The Minister calls for evidence to inform policy decisions. And indeed, a survey was subsequently carried out in collaboration with NAC. However, the report of the survey results—if there was a report—was never circulated (Susan Watkins conversation with Agnes Chimbiri, the director of the survey).

P41 Interview with a Cabinet Minister

Previously Malawi as a nation was a secret nation. A secret in that we didn't have TVs we didn't have videos. We didn't have pornography. We didn't have some of these things they are coming in as new things. So you have certain behaviours and changes that have come in or practices that have come in that were not there. In terms of policy as an office we are now moving where we have already developed a proposal where we want to do a comprehensive study on cultural practices from Nsanje to Chipita for every district. And document them. Having documented them we will form a chiefs' council or a chiefs' committee then we will form the initiators' committee, the traditional birth attendants' committee then we use these committees to identify those who have an education and train them on addressing the cultural practices. So that we identify the good ones that we can use. For example soon after delivery three months must pass before having sexual intercourse.......That's a cultural practice but it is a good one. It allowed the woman to recover fully but at the same time it was protecting against sexually transmitted diseases and the man was told the minute you have sexual intercourse with another woman the child is going to die. And which man was willing to let the child die? You see. There were those. And these are the good cultural practices. So we wanted them in their own set up to identify the good cultural practices the harmful cultural practices and promote the good ones. Let me say not really discard. But let's say modify the harmful ones so that they can work better.

What we see, in districts where HIV was lower, it's a rural district, it's developing quickly and the prevalence is rising. And behind that we know it is the cultural practices. The prevalence in young people, the new prevalence in young people still remains quite high at 18 per cent we know it is because of the cultural practices. So we are more than ready to do the practice but to inform policy. We are not looking at it to inform HIV national response. No. Because this is where our donor partners get confused. When we put out our proposal they will see we are already giving our money. Yeah but NAC is not solving the global issues of Malawi. It is doing work that is looking at coordinating the implementation of the national response. But from the global aspects we have to look at these like er these sociocultural aspects. We can't not just deal with within the closed component we have to look at it from a broader perspective. (P41)

What is clear in in the interview with the Minister above is the direct and over simplified link being made between Harmful Cultural Practices and HIV transmission as well as the assumption that the cultural practices are to blame for the increase in HIV prevalence rates in rural areas.

The P25 interview with a Programme Officer below demonstrates how a Malawian elite is making the assumption that these 'negative' practices take place in rural areas thus distancing herself from the villages and demonstrating her 'eliteness'. It also shows how she thinks the village chiefs are to blame as she says the chief said that they themselves are perpetuating these cultural practices. she says 'stakeholders meet all people who are dealing with women and HIV/AIDS issues'.

P25 Interview with a Programme Officer

Basically, I think there is going to be, I am not sure because there is a consultant that has been hired to give an inception report on how best we can be able to 'cause you know cultural issues the moment you go to the communities and start saying 'ok, we've come here we want to know the negative cultural practices, they are not going to tell you. It's something that is really sort of a secretive thing within the community. Ok, there has to be somebody who is living within the community to be able to, after sometime to be able to get this kind of data. However, we do have some leaders that are coming out openly; we have some chiefs, nowadays, that are really acknowledging that these things are happening. For instance, we have this Kwataine, he is a chief in Ntcheu where the stakeholders meet all people who are dealing with women and HIV/AIDS issues; he actually came out and said 'you know, let's not hide, indeed these things are happening in our communities, and some of them it's even us the chiefs that are perpetuating these cultural practices, so we need to do something about it ourselves. So we just want to get at least some information trying to use focus groups, not focus groups, one on one interviews with the leaders within the communities that are doing initiation ceremonies. Yeah. We want to get their opinion because they are very instrumental in terms of knowing cultural issues, but mmm many are major key players within the community in all sorts of issues. Aah, they are the role models within the communities that we could try get them and try to hear from them; their views. But also the traditional leaders themselves, although they might hide information, sometimes they can slip off the tongue and tell you some stuff. So, we don't want just to interview everybody, you know. (P25)

When I interviewed the District AIDS Coordinator in Balaka he told me that during a proposal writing training, CBO members were asked to mention some of the cultural practices that are practised in their areas. When I asked why he said:

We feel that maybe some of the cultural practices are contributing to the spread of HIV/AIDS. So maybe we want to see if they know that these cultural practices can contribute to the spread of HIV/AIDS, how can they end those cultural practices or how they can tackle those problems. (P13)

Again the oversimplification is clear. I asked him why he felt the need to talk about cultural practices and he laughed. I said is it in your policy or mandate to say I need to ask them about cultural practices? He said we do that just because it's a mandate of the job, it's a mandate of the job to tackle each and every issue that can contribute to HIV/AIDS. I asked him where did his understanding of the issues come from? He didn't understand my question so I rephrased it and said if you think cultural practices contribute to the spread of AIDS, why do you, where have you learnt that they do. He said:

You know, there are some things you don't need to learn, but you can just think and prove yourself that when doing this this can happen, when doing this this can happen. But I will say that I have attended a number of workshops whereby people share experiences and whatsoever, in so doing it's when I have known some of these things. (P13)

When I asked him where he said 'a number of workshops, maybe some of them maybe review meetings conducted by NAC, some of them maybe some of the stakeholders'. I asked him when people talk about the cultural practices which ones do you think are contributing to the spread of AIDS? He said 'maybe the initiation ceremony and *kuchotsa fumbi*, (in *Chichewa* it is *kulowa kufa*)'. I said, how did you hear about these practices. He said:

> Yeah, no no, it's like just because people have been saying much on these cultural practices so that maybe people should stop this. So it's not even maybe to hear without asking, but these policies are been done aaah, down down down down so that maybe a lot of people should not see that people are doing there that just because people have already said no stop this, no stop this. So these are happening but in dark corners. I said so like in secret? He said yeah yeah in secret. (P13)

In interviews with members of the medical profession the hazy understanding of harmful cultural practices was clear. Given how little clear knowledge of harmful cultural practices, prevalence and nature of the practices exist it is further strange that harmful cultural practices have been brought so centrally into policies on AIDS.

I spoke with a director of a small CBO and asked his definition of the *fisi* sexual practice. He told me there is *kutchosa fumbi* and *fisi:*

> 1. *Kutchosa fumbi* – Initiation ceremony. Give counselling to young girls who have just grown up to give them advice and how they can live with elders and the like. Sometimes they do advise them to have sexual intercourse with the boys in the villages. So it's like to see if they can have pregnancies and a child. It's like to test/check if they can have a child. After that ceremony they get boys or men to have sexual intercourse with those young girls. The girls are aged 12-18. 2. *Fisi* – You get married, man is failing in home to have a child. So you consult another man so he can have a child within the family. It's a consultation issue. It is not usually ladies but men sometimes. (Journal entry, 11 November 2008)

INITIATION

Subsequently, UNFPA conducted a survey in Malawi (and in other countries) to assess the problem of harmful cultural practices called Safeguarding Young People Programme: Cultural Practices Study (UNFPA 2015). UNFPA-Malawi's Call for Proposals for this study stated "most of the cultural initiation ceremonies that young people are expressed to violate their rights and are risky and a form of abuse" (UNFPA 2015, p. 6). This study is important and resonates

4 'HARMFUL CULTURAL PRACTICES' AND AIDS

Table 4.1 Received information on the following topics at initiation

Content of information	Overall N=283 N (%)	Males N=98 N (%)	Females N=185 N (%)	P-value
Growing up and changes in the body for girls	152 (53.7)	39 (39.8)	113 (61.1)	**<0.001**
Growing up and changes in body for boys	115 (40.6)	45 (45.9)	70 (37.8)	0.2
Sexual feelings and emotions	112 (39.6)	33 (33.7)	79 (42.7)	0.1
Sexual intercourse	75 (26.5)	25 (25.5)	50 (27.0)	0.7
Conception	21 (7.4)	2 (2.0)	19 (10.3)	**0.01**
Pregnancy	76 (26.9)	7 (7.1)	69 (37.3)	**<0.001**
Child birth	24 (8.5)	2 (2.0)	22 (11.9)	**0.004**
Being a parent	24 (8.5)	1 (1.0)	23 (12.4)	**0.001**
Contraception	43 (15.2)	5 (5.1)	38 (20.5)	**<0.0001**
Safe sex	42 (14.8)	10 (10.2)	32 (17.3)	0.1
Sexually transmitted infections	97 (34.3)	24 (24.5)	73 (39.5)	**0.009**
HIV/AIDS	107 (37.8)	25 (25.5)	82 (44.3)	**0.001**
Respecting elders	80 (28.3)	30 (30.6)	50 (27.1)	0.6

* Percentages calculated using the total number of subjects who participated in initiation ceremonies; statistically significant differences in bold

Table 4.2 New knowledge provided during initiation ceremony

Type of information	Felt the information provided during the initiation ceremony was different from what already knew			
	Total initiated N=283 N (%)	Males, N=98 N (%)	Females, N=185 N (%)	P-value
Growing up and changes in the body for girls	62 (21.9)	18 (18.4)	44 (23.8)	0.3
Growing up and changes in body for boys	52 (18.4)	16 (16.3)	36 (19.5)	0.5
Sexual feelings and emotions	59 (20.9)	19 (19.4)	40 (21.6)	0.6
Sexual intercourse	28 (9.9)	6 (6.1)	22 (11.9)	0.1
Conception	10 (3.5)	1 (1.0)	9 (4.9)	0.09
Pregnancy	39 (13.8)	9 (9.2)	30 (16.2)	0.1
Child birth	14 (5.0)	2 (2.0)	12 (6.5)	0.1
Being a parent	11 (4.0)	2 (2.0)	9 (4.9)	0.2
Contraception	38 (13.4)	8 (8.2)	30 (16.2)	**0.05**
Safe sex	17 (6.0)	3 (3.1)	14 (7.6)	0.1
Sexually transmitted infections	55 (19.4)	15 (15.3)	40 (21.6)	0.2
HIV/AIDS	57 (20.1)	17 (17.4)	40 (21.6)	0.4
Respecting elders	59 (20.9)	24 (24.5)	35 (18.9)	0.3

*Percentages calculated using the total number of subjects who participated in initiation ceremonies; statistically significant differences in bold

Table 4.3 List of items liked during initiation ceremonies

Type of activity	N (%)
Gained new knowledge	45 (15.9)
Trained to respect elders	34 (12.0)
Dances	18 (6.4)
Good food	16 (5.7)
Being circumcised	15 (5.3)
Given new clothes at the end of the ceremony	13 (4.6)
Safe sex education	12 (4.2)
Not afraid/belonging to *nyau*	11 (3.9)
Made new friends	11 (3.9)
Given money at the end of the ceremony	9 (3.2)
Learned about their culture	8 (2.8)
Learned how to take care of themselves during menstruation	7 (2.5)
Sex education	5 (1.8)
Gained respect in the community after attending the ceremony	5 (1.8)
Trained on abstinence	5 (1.8)
Happy to attend the ceremony	5 (1.8)
Well taken care of by initiator during the ceremony	4 (1.4)
Was allowed access to other initiation sites after the ceremony	3 (1.1)
Attendance resulted in change of behavior	3 (0.4)
Gained sense of belonging because friends had already attended the ceremony	2 (0.7)
Learned about body development	2 (0.7)
Obtained more information on HIV	1 (0.4)
Taught to work hard at school	1 (0.4)
The advice was similar to what was learnt at school	1 (0.4)
They followed the rules of Islamic teaching	1 (0.4)
Was not beaten or slapped	1 (0.4)
Was the youngest and was therefore getting a lot of attention	1 (0.4)
Liked the way the advice was given	1 (0.4)

*Percentages calculated using the total number of subjects who participated in initiation ceremonies

with my findings as it shows that it was precisely because UNFPA at the international and national level belived that girls suffered from sexual cultural practices that the study was carried out. However this study found that central to inititation is to transition to adulthood. The core of the initiation is to learn how to be an adult: adult advisers tell the initiates what they should and should not do now that they are adults. In Tables 4.1, 4.2, 4.3 and 4.4 we see that children looked forward to the initiation and *fisi* were never mentioned. Virtually all were pleased with initiation—the man reason for liking the cerermony

Table 4.4 List of activities not liked during initiation ceremonies

Type of activity	Overall N= 112[a] N (%)
Beating/bullying	28 (22.4)
Obscene language used during the ceremony and in songs	17 (12.8)
Being forced to have sex after the initiation ceremony	14 (11.2)
Long duration	11 (8.8)
Being naked during the ceremony	5 (4.0)
Songs and dance	5 (4.0)
Pain following circumcision	4 (3.2)
Rudeness of initiators	4 3.2)
Too much sex information	4 (3.2)
Early wake up time	4 (3.2)
Being smeared with mud	2 (1.6)
Told not to chat with boys	2 (1.6)
Being asked to dig a pit to be buried alive	1 (0.8)
Cold bathing water	1 (0.8)
Dropping out of school	1 (0.8)
Not being given food	1 (0.8)
Late bedtime	1 (0.8)
Not given detailed education information	1 (0.8)
Asked to drink medicine	1 (0.8)
Not allowed to bath	1 (0.8)
Stealing	1 (0.8)
Exposing young children to sex information	1 (0.8)
Told to get married	1 (0.8)
Was advised while too young	1 (0.8)

[a] N is number of responses, not number of respondents. Respondents could give more than one answer
*Percentages calculated using the total number of subjects who participated in initiation; the categories are not mutually exclusive

was that initiates learned something new (UNFPA 2015, p. 39). Girls liked receiving new information about menstruation and sexual health. When asked what they didn't like it was activities such as beating/bullying, the ceremony took too long, bad language used during ceremony or songs, or having to bathe in cold water during the days of seclusion (for girls). And, while occassionally a *fisi* may be called for initiation, it was not frequent enough to be mentioned in the survey responses, even to the questions about "What did you not like about the initiation ceremonies?" (Table 4.5).

Table 4.5 Negative experiences during the initiation ceremonies by age

Type of negative experience	Number of initiates N=283 N (%)	10–14 years, N=77	15–19 years, N=116	20–24 years, N=88	P-value
Forced touching (genitals, breasts or buttocks)	46 (16.3)	12 (15.6)	19 (16.4)	15 (17.1)	0.9
Forced sex (penetrative, non-penetrative)	10 (3.5)	2 (2.6)	5 (4.3)	3 (3.4)	0.8
Forced oral sex	7 (2.5)	2 (2.6)	3 (2.6)	2 (2.3)	0.9
Forced exposure to sex	30 (10.6)	6 (7.8)	13 (11.2)	11 (12.4)	0.6
Forced exposure to sex materials	16 (5.7)	3 (3.9)	6 (5.2)	7 (8.0)	0.5
Bullying	53 (18.7)	13 (16.9)	20 (17.2)	20 (22.7)	0.5
Slapped/beaten/pinched	89 (31.5)	24 (31.2)	40 (24.5)	25 (28.4)	0.7
Denied food	26 (9.2)	6 (7.8)	6 (5.2)	14 (15.9)	**0.03**
Others (forced to dance while naked)	1 (0.4)	1 (1.3)	0	0	0.5

*Percentages calculated using the total number of subjects who participated in initiation ceremonies including missing values

Narratives of Blame Among the Malawian Elite: 'Rural Communities as Backwards'

This section demonstrates how people I interviewed perceive rural villagers as backwards and how those that live in rural areas are to blame for the spread of HIV. For example, a lawyer said:

> So you find that in cases where a man and woman want to engage in sexual intercourse, you find that the woman is so powerless; as a matter of fact you don't question what a man wants to do, especially for the rural folk. (P26)

Whereas the respondent suggests there is a gender imbalance in sexual relationships she places particular emphasis on the rural population. The 'rural folk' are especially to blame for gender imbalances—blaming the rural male in particular for sexual dominance and reinforcing the stereotype of the sexually, virile village man and the powerless rural, woman.

P15 Interview with a District Youth Officer

R: These cultural practices were revealed by the community members themselves; they said yes, these are the cultural practices which we feel are contributing to HIV.

S: Do you think it will be a problem, a big problem or a small problem or –

R: When we look at cultural issues usually it can be simple but for those which, for the Balaka district here, I understand these are very big problems.

S: Why?

R: Aaah, you know cultural issues are regarded as very very important behaviour in a village setting.

S: Ok.

R: So they can't go away with those unless we have to change some of the cultural issues, not to completely put them out but just change them so that at least they should be friendly to the women.

S: How will you...?

R: Aaah, as a district, first of all our aim is to enlighten the community on these cultural issues, because they have been with these cultural issues since time immemorial.

S: Yah.

R: So we have to tell them, we enlighten them as to why, we say that these cultural issues are exposing women to HIV/AIDS. They have been doing these things since time in memorial, so they don't know it is there, but when you enlighten them it is for them to think that oh no we need to change our behaviour.

S: Do you think they will change their behaviour as a result of you discussing?

R: Changing behaviour is a slow process, so we hope with our continued information on these issues they are going to change.

S: Key issue in Balaka, I mean in terms of HIV prevalence rate? What do you think is the main problem as regard to HIV/AIDS in Balaka? Is it cultural practices or is it something else?

R: You know cultural practices are there, but we can say there are so many things. The other side we are looking at cultural practices, but we also have to look at the behaviour of the community.

S: Yeah, So how are you looking at them?

R: Aaah, when I look at the behaviour of the community, the behaviour of the community around, in townships yeah; usually in townships we have all those people who are going out, they don't have money and what. But I don't know, I think we should say, for the things which are, because I have to say things which I have seen myself.

S: Sure.

R: I can not say I have seen people doing that and that because these are the things which are
S: Ok.
R: Yeah.
S: Like you said, cultural practices, you haven't seen them happen?
R: Aah I should say yes but the people themselves, because these issues were given to me by the traditional authorities, they said they are happening in the villages.
S: And these aah, these traditional authorities, they want them to change, do they want to change?
R: Yeah.
S: They said that to you?
R: Yeah, they want to change because when we have given them the questions which are which are the cultural issues, you would see that they are contributing to HIV/AIDS. And I said what do you think this could be changed or what do you think we can reduce HIV/AIDS looking at those cultural issues; I think it's also highlighted on the paper. I've already said that behavioural change is a slow process; we need to still enlighten them more so that at least they have to change. (P15)

The District Officer attended a technical college in Malawi. He told me about sexual cultural practices taking place and blamed people living in rural areas. He said that sexual cultural practices are taking place in the district of Balaka that are spreading HIV. He also says that although he has never seen a practice take place he has been told about them by the traditional authorities. This point highlights once again how people working on AIDS report that the practice takes place even though they have never witnessed it themselves thus perpetuating the misconception concerning the link between sexual cultural practices and AIDS.

The following is an excerpt from an interview carried out with a midwife working at Balaka District Hospital. She has a nursing degree.

P8 Interview with a Midwife

Ok, so I will just ask some questions about the cultural practices. Maybe you could just tell me if your, like what cultural practices take place in Balaka that you say you are aware of that might contribute to the spread of HIV/AIDS?

R: Yeah. The ones I'm aware of it's like kusasa fumbi, and this kusasa fumbi it's after the girls have been, after the –
S: Yah.

R: Then they go to, they say chinamwali where are being taught how they can maybe play sex with the men, then after that they are told to practice.
S: Ok.
R: So they take just any other person.
S: Yah.
R: Yah.
S: So when does this cultural practice take place, what do you think or know?
R: Aah, I don't know much but, you mean in terms of months or –
S: Yah.
R: Most of the times it's during the dry season.
S: Yah, ok. So probably between, around I don't know, May?
R: I think around July, August, September, these months.
S: Ok. And do you hear about the cultural practices much or not really? I mean in terms of your work, is it an issue for you?
R: Yah, of course we hear because we usually know them when they go into the street singing from the chinamwali site.
S: But in terms of, do you hear in your work?
R: No.
S: No one mentions it?
R: Mmhmm.
S: So maybe it's not quite a big issue regarding the prevalence rate of HIV/AIDS, it's not something that really, do you think it's a big issue in terms of spreading HIV/AIDS?
R: Yah, it is. Because around the town we can not say much but when you go into the villages that's when you see a lot of people practising those.
S: Ok, do you think it's in most areas?
R: Yah, it is in most areas because this area is full of the Islam they are the ones who practise these a lot than other tribes. (P8)

In a training manual produced by Oxfam and SAFAIDS entitled 'Interlinkages Between Culture, Gender-based Violence, HIV/AIDS and Women's Rights' it states: 'This training manual seeks to make development agents aware that there is not much that can be achieved in the response to HIV/AIDS if society does not deal with the root cause of the problem – CULTURE' (SafAIDS 2008, p. 5). The manual's cover depicts a photo of African women and men singing and dressed in informal attire, which suggests they are from a rural area. The manual was developed for use by community workers and volunteers, HIV/AIDS programmers and programme implementers, CBOs and FBOs and provides a step-by-step guide on how to run a four-day workshop and includes hand-outs.

The manual goes on to talk about 'the role of culture in HIV prevention'.

Culture is important for understanding the HIV/AIDS epidemic in sub-Saharan Africa. It helps to explain, in part, the high HIV/AIDS prevalence rates, particularly among women. Numerous cultural beliefs and practices, such as wife/husband inheritance, polygamy, spirit appeasement, lack of communication about sexual matters between men and women, gender inequity and culturally-sanctioned extramarital affairs and infidelity among men, have been tied to the high rates of STIs including HIV. (SAfAIDS 2008, p. 26)

This manual ignores epidemiological evidence and blames cultural practices for high HIV prevalence rates. The manual also provides a handout which lists eight negative cultural practices that are linked to gender and HIV. Such manuals imply that culture is negative. ActionAid's country strategy paper 2005–2010 also makes reference to 'negative cultural practices' (2005, p. 13). These manuals also contradict global policy documents linked between cultural practices and gender-based violence which is very confusing.

DISTORTION OF THE REALITY

As mentioned the actual risk of HIV infection from one act of heterosexual intercourse is 1 in 1000 (Gray et al. 2001). However, what is interesting is that many Malawians believe that HIV is easily transmitted. In several surveys conducted in a research project, the MDICP, which look at the role of social networks in influencing responses to the AIDS epidemic in rural Malawi, respondents were asked how likely it was that one act of sexual intercourse with an HIV infected person would lead to infection for the other partner. More than 95% said the probability of transmission was either certain or highly likely (Watkins and Swidler 2009).

Furthermore, ethnographic journals recorded by Malawian high school graduates who wrote down anything they overheard concerning AIDS—what Watkins and Swidler (2009) refers to as 'hearsay ethnography' revealed that Malawians come to the conclusion that if a person has had sex with someone who is already infected then that person will also be infected: 'Thus, when a young man says, after his first sexual encounter with a young woman who he hopes will be his "real girlfriend," that "Indeed, friend, if Grace has AIDS, she has given it to me, I couldn't resist her attractions"' (Simon 2001, cited by Watkins and Swidler 2009, p. 442).

In another excerpt the point above is made again in that if a husband is infected then the wife must be and vice versa:

> She said, 'Yes indeed, people say that lying together is dying together. If he has HIV/AIDS, I have HIV/AIDS but I know that we don't have it'.
>
> And I asked, 'How do you know? Did you go for a blood test?'
>
> She said, 'I know myself and he told me one day that he doesn't have HIV/AIDS. He went for a blood test and found that he doesn't have it' (Simon, 2001, cited by Watkins et al. 2011, p. 442). These points reaffirm my argument concerning Malawians' claims that HIV is easily transmitted through heterosexual intercourse.

A lawyer asserted: 'let me tell you this thing of us, men want to have sexual intercourse with younger women because they believe that they are virgins and therefore they don't have HIV' (P26).

P36 Interview with a Policy Advisor

> R: Because you know culture, culture in Malawi is so... it's something that leads to many problems; it leads to many problems. And when we talk about culture you need to break it down. Because even raping of children, small children is out of belief, out of cultural belief that say maybe when you sleep with a six-month-old baby you get healed of HIV/AIDS. So I'm looking at culture as something that has brought more harm than good in terms of upholding people's identity or you know...
>
> S: Do you really think that happens?
>
> R: You mean raping children? Ahh!
>
> S: Really?
>
> R: Really... it's rampant. (P36)

The country director of Trocaire holds a diploma in development management. He told me that Trocaire was looking to conduct:

> Cultural research linked to HIV and women's vulnerability, for example women that sell sex for fish. To do a good piece of solid research – and look at aspects of that vulnerability – why are men so stark? Why do they have to have 3-4 wives? Cultural stuff – some believe that during harvest of fish they need to have sex with someone else. Useful for advocacy and furthering other projects (P27)

And as a Minister explained:

> This was the truth and then we formed a technical subcommittee because there were a lot of technical communication which was about condoms and the small holes there and the rubber and the virus is smaller and it can go through so how so we wanted to correct this technical misinformation. But I must say that since then there have been improvements and they have formed their own organisation called the Malawi Interfaith Aids Association (MIAA) (P5).

Conclusion

In this chapter I have shown that Malawian elites' view is that cultural practices are harmful (from policy documents, interviews and newspapers). The epidemiology of the virus contradicts their views that transmission probability is low. The elite blame rural people for the high HIV prevalence rates, pinpointing their cultural practices described as backward and contrasted against their own enlightened status.

The 'harmful' side of these practices is an 'imagined fact' in terms of how they contribute to high prevalence rates but also in terms of where they are observed. It was clear that the Malawian elite knew relatively little about harmful cultural practices, and where they were practiced. The inconsistencies and inaccuracy in the explanations given serve as further evidence that a narrative of blame has clearly been constructed that seeks to pin blame on rural communities and a set of 'backward' beliefs. Furthermore, there is a disconnect between the educated elite and rural villagers. The elite distance themselves so blame other sections of society, particularly those that live in rural areas. They do not just blame a cultural practice but portray these communities as being backward as they want to maintain their own image on a par with international donors. I also looked at where their perception of harmful cultural practices comes from and the motivation for holding them.

All Malawian respondents are elite, live in urban areas and want to disassociate with Malawi's image of a very poor country, they do this by contrasting themselves against rural villagers who they claim to be backward and not like them. Very few of them have lived in a rural village so they would not have any first-hand knowledge about the harmful cultural practices, they may know the names of a few practices from their grandparents in the villages, but that's it. The educated elite in general are religious, Christian, their religion, the result of conversion during the missionary phase of Malawi's history, has become for them an identifying mark of their developed enlightened status. Their Christian beliefs contrasted against the traditional practices of the rural 'other' who remains uncivilised and unenlightened. I also argued that a further motive exists for maintaining these narratives of blame. They secure longer term positions for those elites awarded responsibilities for eradicating them. In the next chapter I delve deeper into the role Christianity has placed in shaping these narratives of blame.

Notes

1. I have been unable to find an English translation for the practices in bold after consulting many Malawians living in Malawi who work on HIV prevention.
2. Interestingly a footnote has been included in the original report which states "similar practices may be known by different names or have derivatives which may not be listed here. It is for this reason that the Minister has been empowered to amend the list as needs arises" (Malawi Law Commission 2008, p. 35). Further, the report did not provide translations so I attempted to provide them.
3. When respondents say most, they don't distinguish between most and many. When they want to say many, they say most, implying almost all.

References

Government of Malawi. (2003). *National HIV/AIDS Policy*. Lilongwe: Malawi.
Gray, R. H., Wawer, M. J., Brookmeyer, R., Sewankambo, N. K., Serwadda, D., Wabwire-Mangen, F., ... & Quinn, T. C. (2001). Probability of HIV-1 transmission per coital act in monogamous, heterosexual, HIV-1-discordant couples in Rakai, Uganda. *The Lancet, 357*(9263), 1149–1153.
Malawi. National Statistical Office, & ICF Macro (Firm). (2011). *Malawi Demographic and Health Survey, 2010*. National Statistical Office.
Malawi Law Commission. (2008). *Report of the Law Commission on the development of HIV and AID legislation*. Lilongwe: Malawi.
MDICP. (2004). *Malawi Diffusion and Ideational Change Project*.
Mkandawire-Valhmu, L., Wendland, C., Stevens, P. E., Kako, P. M., Dressel, A., & Kibicho, J. (2013). Marriage as a risk factor for HIV: Learning from the experiences of HIV-infected women in Malawi. *Global Public Health, 8*(2), 187–201.

Morfit, N. S. (2011). "AIDS is money": How donor preferences reconfigure local realities. *World Development, 39*(1), 64–76.

Myroniuk, T. W. (2011). Global discourses and experiential speculation: Secondary and tertiary graduate Malawians dissect the HIV/AIDS epidemic. *Journal of the International AIDS Society, 14*(1), 47.

SafAIDS. (2008). *Inter-linkages between culture, gender based violence, HIV/AIDS and women's rights: Training manual.* Zimbabwe: SAfAIDS.

Swidler, A., & Watkins, S. C. (2009). "Teach a man to fish": The sustainability doctrine and its social consequences. *World Development, 37*(7), 1182–1196.

Swidler, A., & Watkins, S. C. (2017). *A fraught embrace: The romance and reality of AIDS altruism in Africa.* Princeton: Princeton University Press.

UN. (1993, December 20). *Declaration on the elimination of violence against women.* A/RES/48/104 85th plenary meeting.

UN. (2000). *Resolution A/RES/54/133 adopted by the General Assembly: Traditional or customary practices affecting the health of women and girls.* Retrieved November 6, 2013, from http://www1.uneca.org/Portals/ngm/Documents/Conventions%20and%20Resolutions/Resolution%20on%20traditional.pdf.

UN. (2011). *Political declaration on HIV and AIDS: Intensifying Our efforts to eliminate HIV and AIDS.* New York: UN.

UN. (2012). *Report of the Secretary General United to end AIDS: Achieving the targets of the 2011 political declaration.* New York: UN.

UN Commission on Human Rights. (2003). *Commission on Human Rights Resolution 2003/45: Elimination of violence against women.* Retrieved November 6, 2013, from the Refworld website http://www.refworld.org/docid/43f3133b0.html.

UNAIDS. (2004). *Malawi country report.* Geneva, Switzerland: UNAIDS.

UNESCO. (2001). *A cultural approach to HIV/AIDS prevention and care.* UNESCO inter-regional conference, 2–4 October 2000, Nairobi, Kenya.

UNFPA. (2013). *Gender equality.* Retrieved October 13, 2013, from http://www.unfpa.org/gender/violence.htm.

UNFPA. (2015). *Safeguard young people: Cultural practices study.* UNFPA-Malawi.

United Nations Malawi. (2008). Agenda Item 56: Advancement of Women to the Third Committee, 63rd session of the United Nations General Assembly, New York 2008, Retrieved November 20, 2018, from http://www.un.org/womenwatch/daw/documents/ga63/malawi.pdf.

Watkins, S. C. (2010). Back to basics: Gender, social norms, and the AIDS epidemic in sub-Saharan Africa. *The Socioeconomic Dimensions of HIV/AIDS in Africa,* 134–162.

Watkins, S. C., & Swidler, A. (2009). Hearsay ethnography: Conversational journals as a method for studying culture in action. *Poetics (Hague, Netherlands), 37*(2), 162.

Watkins, S. C., Swidler, A., & Biruk, C. (2011). Hearsay ethnography: A method for learning about responses to health interventions. In *Handbook of the sociology of health, illness, and healing* (pp. 431–445). New York: Springer.

Open Access This chapter is licensed under the terms of the Creative Commons Attribution 4.0 International License (http://creativecommons.org/licenses/by/4.0/), which permits use, sharing, adaptation, distribution and reproduction in any medium or format, as long as you give appropriate credit to the original author(s) and the source, provide a link to the Creative Commons licence and indicate if changes were made.

The images or other third party material in this chapter are included in the chapter's Creative Commons licence, unless indicated otherwise in a credit line to the material. If material is not included in the chapter's Creative Commons licence and your intended use is not permitted by statutory regulation or exceeds the permitted use, you will need to obtain permission directly from the copyright holder.

CHAPTER 5

How the Church Frames AIDS

Religious Context in Malawi

Malawi is a very religious country; around 77% of the population is Christian, 15% Muslim and 8% practice traditional African religions (Barrett et al. 2001). Among the Christians, 25% are Roman Catholics, 20% are Protestants and 17% are members of African Independent Churches. Evangelicals and Pentecostals are on the increase, particularly in urban areas, and together account for about 32% (Jenkins 2011). Evangelicals and Pentecostals are less numerous in rural areas than in urban areas, and Muslims are largely concentrated in the South of the country. These figures are estimates and are provided by national denominational organisations rather than based on representative surveys of national populations and therefore may be incorrect (Trinatopoli 2006).

Gathering data on religious affiliation is further complicated by the syncretic nature of religion in Malawi which results in hybrid religious groups that might not reflect denominational characteristics as in other parts of Africa. In Malawi, Christianity and traditional religion are often combined (P44). This means that the line between Christianity and tradition is often blurred and African conceptions of politics and religion do not always separate the Church from the State (Patterson 2011, p. 3).

A Member of Parliament told me:

> But after Christianity, there has been another level of Christianity which is the, they call themselves the indigenous Christian churches. They are Christians but they have taken aspects of the Chewa tradition and said no no, we have we have our own way of looking at God's revelation but they emphasise a lot on the Bible and I am not an expert on that but I can tell you about the Chewa traditional religion. One God, monotheistic, that one is really highly developed and when you read it and you look at Christianity there is hardly much difference, but the way the Christians, the missionaries came, they had to demonise it, that this is primitive; it's not the right way of looking at religion but actually no, they believed in one God and called him different names but who doesn't call God different names? The Jews call him all kinds of names, the Christians call him all kinds of names, why should the Chewa not call it that, because God showed all his power in different forms. And they called ours ancestral spirit worship, no, they never worshipped the spirits. They looked at the spirits as intercessors to God, God was looked at as the supreme spirit. When you die you become a spirit, so you are nearer God so you can communicate better with God so you pray to God straight, directly, and then afterwards you call upon your ancestors to intercede for you, to pray for you. The Christians also do the same and now pray for Mary, what are they, are they alive, they are dead (laughter). So actually you can go through the tradition, the Chewa traditional religion quite similarly, I wish they had understood it and then say yes this is how you believe, it is quite correct, but the transformation of your belief into Jesus as the universal saviour, that would have gone very well with the Chewa. But they said stop, no, once you become a Christian, you stop everything. And that to my mind, and I am a Christian, my father was a Christian, but I think a lot of Malawians have really, are not what we say we are, because they can't take this out of us, they can't, we are still a Chewa. (P5)

Here we see a divide between those that combine African Traditional Religion (ATR) with Christianity and those that only practise Christian beliefs. The elite perceives themselves as such because they have rejected

ATR in favour of Christianity as taught by the missionaries. This illustrates how a divide has emerged internally to Malawi and how this has, in turn, shaped the perceptions the elite have of the rural populations who they see as backward because they still practice traditional religion so to be enlightened is to reject tradition. ATR is difficult to define primarily because it is lived and not preached and followers are preoccupied with the practice of ATR rather than theory; therefore there is no single, simple and precise definition to describe it. Mbiti (1970) provides a useful summary of where to look for and find ATR. He suggests rituals, ceremonies and festivals; shrines, sacred places and religious objects; art and symbols; music and dance; proverbs, riddles and wise sayings; names of people and places; myths and legends and beliefs and customs. Bascom and Herskovits (1962, p. 3) argued that despite the intensity of Christian missionary efforts and the thousand years of Muslim proselytising which have marked parts of Africa, ATRs continued to manifest everywhere. This was seen in the worship of African deities, the homage to ancestors and the recourse to divination, magic and other rituals.

Using broad categories of African Christian churches provided by Gifford (2004, p. 10), the estimated number of Christians categorised by churches in Malawi at the time (2001) with a population of 10.9 million was: Orthodox 4400; Catholics 2.7 million; Old Mission Protestants (Mainlines) 2.37 million; New Mission Protestants (Faith-Mission and Pentecostals) 130,000; Old Independents (African Indigenous) 2 million; and New Independents (neo-Pentecostals and Charismatics) 1.46 million (Barrett et al. 2001). As we can see from these figures, Catholicism is the most popular type of Christianity with New Mission Protestants the least popular with a large percentage of the population still practising traditional religion. As this paragraph demonstrates there are many different types of Christianity in Malawi and within each type, variations exist. For example, Pentecostals vary greatly and many congregations may have local autonomy from other churches but there can be a considerable hierarchy within individual organisations (Patterson 2011, p. 79).

However, as we have seen through my interviews there is an overlap between ATR and Christianity. The idea of 'divine punishment' is common to ATR and Christianity and resonates with 'transgressing taboos' (Lwanda 2005, p. 120). Some Christians, although criticising cultural practices for spreading HIV, accepted 'conservative' or formative aspects of ATR. Lwanda (2005) makes the link between medicine and Christianity and ATR and posits the view that in rural and peri-urban areas, disagreements between Christianity and western medicine and ATR and traditional medicine were solved by cultural dualities as opposed to hybridity or cultural subjugation (Lwanda 2005, p. 83). He argues that:

> Many core cultural beliefs, now embedded in village localities, were not significantly challenged by colonial or Christian assaults; they had been placed out of the colonial gaze. The invisibility often gave the impression of, and was mistaken for, indigenous practices dying out under the over-whelming and inhibitory nature of colonial governance. Dualism enabled many Maravai to survive colonialism without experiencing 'dissolution' or 'fragmentation' (mental illnesses resulting from cultural alienation or maladjustment) (Fanon, 1970, p. 7 and p. 77) a more common experience among educated elite who, unlike the more culturally secure villagers, had to confront the cultural dichotomy head on. (p. 84)

Patterson makes a similar point but related to the use of anti-retroviral drugs. She points out that while some churches are suspicious of ARVs, God can be the only true healer. Some churches then combine the use of ARVs with spiritual healing (Patterson 2011). However pastors may also use prayer, exorcism, fasting or traditional herbs to drive the virus from the believer's body (Becker and Geissler 2007, p. 11). This example shows how a tension exists between spiritual and biomedical approaches to treatment.

District Interfaith AIDS Committees (DIACS) exist in Malawi and there are 32 in total, comprising 12 members from different churches at district levels. The DIAC nominates a chairperson, secretary and treasurer to run the committee. At the district level, activities for faith-based HIV/AIDS programmes take place which are run through the local churches of each faith group. The Malawi Interfaith AIDS Association (MIAA) has trained all DIACs and have linked them to the District Assembly. Religious leadership is generally male, although some of the evangelical Malawi churches are led by women but the wider social structures they promote are still patriarchal despite a female figurehead. The Protestant and Roman Catholic churches focus on behaviours—fidelity and abstinence, for instance—as a means to prevent STIs; in other words, the focus is placed on the maintenance of a heterosexual status quo with emphasis placed on women as the homemakers and child rearers as the model most likely to see low infection rates. However, some critics think focusing on behaviour change alone, rather than changing its context, results in bad policy decisions (Barnett and Parkhurst 2005).

A study by Trinitapoli (2009) examined religious teachings and influences on the Abstain, Be Faithful, use a Condom (ABC) approach of HIV prevention in Malawi. She presents an overview of the topics religious leaders in rural Malawi formally address in their weekly religious services. Over 88% of religious leaders reported preaching about morality (generally); and over 70% preaching about sexual morality; AIDS and illness (generally). Furthermore, 95% of religious leaders reported that they advise their members privately to stop promiscuity yet only 27% reported talking to members on an individual basis about the use of condoms (Trinitapoli 2009, p. 203). Religious leaders generally tend to be male. Some evangelical churches in Malawi are led by women, but the wider social structures they foster are still patriarchal despite having a female leader (Rankin et al. 2006). Soothill's research examined women's empowerment in Ghana's Charismatic Churches (Soothill 2011). During her fieldwork, participating in women's activities of three charismatic churches in Accra, she discovered that in contrast to Ghana's older mission-style churches (predominantly Catholic, Methodist and Presbyterian), the charismatic churches embrace the concept of women's leadership and cast aside traditional barriers to women becoming pastors and church founders. Although the ratio of female to male pastors is still low and the men still dominate the movement in practice, the 'spiritual equality' of believers is a cornerstone of the charismatic discourse on gender (p. 84). Soothill goes on to say however that women in position of religious leadership has not reversed patriarchy.

I collected newspaper articles on HIV/AIDS spanning 10 years during my fieldwork such as the one presented above. Many of them conveyed negative messages concerning AIDS and that condoms are 'useless things' and how everyone 'should kneel before God in order to be protected'. This viewpoint, from a biomedical and feminist viewpoint, is dangerous as it ignores the social reality of male sexual behaviour. The heavy emphasis in religious and public discourse on the importance of women as nurturers fails to acknowledge that the problem predominantly lies in the construction of masculinity that associates sexual prowess with a hyper-masculinity that in turn is desired (Gilmore 1990). A concept of religious morality has clearly been employed in these advertisements. Such messages clearly deny that male promiscuity is both normalised but also legitimised by and through hegemonic constructions of male behaviour. Such religious beliefs ironically promote unprotected sex and have been considered to hamper HIV prevention programmes (Caldwell et al. 1999).

Gama (2000) reported that Malawi's Council of Churches condemn the distribution and use of condoms to prevent HIV transmission as immoral since the government's doing so is tantamount to supporting promiscuity. According to the Church in Malawi, condoms are not 100% effective in preventing infection, noting that the only way to protect oneself is strict monogamy or abstinence. Church leaders make it clear that although non-governmental organisations (NGOs) distribute condoms, they will not distribute or condone their use. This widespread antipathy to condom use has not helped discordant couples, nor has the occasional policy of requiring HIV blood tests before marriage and then refusing to marry discordant couples. A study by Kaler (2004) of the percentage distribution of themes in negative evaluations of condoms in Malawi showed that 16% ($n=7$) reported that using condoms is against God's will. Religion clearly influences people's behaviour and Chaves (2002) suggests three types of religious organisations are thought to influence the behaviour of individuals: congregations, denominational organisations and religious non-profit organisations. However, there are more than three. Churches are often seen as civil society actors and in the 1900s, donors and scholars were looking for agents of political change and socioeconomic development that were independent of the perceived corrupt and inefficient African state (Bratton 1989; Harbeson et al. 1994; Gifford 1998; Patterson 2011). Furthermore, the problems with structural adjustment policies led Africans to identify new alternatives to the state for services, such as religious organisations (Jenkins 2007). According to the Gallup News Service (2007) religious organisations are the most trusted organisations in African civil society due to their links with communities, with 76% of respondents in nineteen countries in sub-Saharan Africa saying they had most confidence in these groups, followed by the military (61%) and financial institutions (55%). They had least confidence in their governments (44%). Gallup further reported that channelling foreign aid through local religious organisations would bring more optimism to African citizens than channelling it directly through the government.

There has been an increase in donor interest and funding of religious groups in development and donors have paid more attention to religion since the United Nations Declaration on HIV/AIDS in 2001 at the General Assembly Special Session on HIV/AIDS. The Declaration mentioned in the previous chapter refers to 'religious factors' that are imperative for HIV prevention and that faith-based organisations provide important leadership in the fight against AIDS (UNAIDS 2001). Dominant donors have taken different approaches. For example, the USA under the Bush administration, approached the issue from a conservative right's view and adopted the ABC approach which echoes the Church in Malawi; that abstinence and monogamy are the only way to reduce AIDS. Perhaps this is why the USA does not put money in the basket funds in Malawi but established the US President's Emergency Plan for AIDS Relief (PEPFAR) and adopted the ABC method as its primary prevention strategy against the sexual transmission of HIV, focusing on Abstinence for youth, including the delay of sexual debut and abstinence until marriage; Being tested for HIV and being faithful in marriage and monogamous relationships and Correct and consistent use of condoms for those who practise high-risk behaviours. This is in contrast to the British government's approach and was one of the main differences between the UK and the USA concerning funding AIDS programmes. DFID adopted the Sector Wide Approach (SWAp), which is supported by a group of development partners and comprises a mix of projects, pooled funding and sector budget support. There is no official definition of the SWAp but it usually adheres to the following:

- All significant funding agencies support a shared, sector-wide policy and strategy, which has clear sector targets and is focused on results;
- A medium-term expenditure framework (MTEF) or budget supports this policy;
- Government provides leadership in a sustained partnership;
- Shared processes and approaches for implementing and managing the sector strategy and work programme are agreed, including reviewing sectoral performance against jointly agreed milestones and targets; and
- There is a shared commitment to move to greater reliance on Government financial management and accountability systems. (Pearson 2010, p. 13)

Since the establishment of the SWAp, DFID has increasingly provided support through Sector Budget Support (SBS) and General Budget Support (GBS) instruments as well as funding service delivery projects off-budget, but under the SWAp which are Banja La Mtsogolo (BLM), which provides family planning and sexual and reproductive health services in a Joint Financing Agreement with Government and other donors; and Voluntary Services Overseas (VSO) which manages a large volunteer programme (Pearson 2010).

Catholic opposition helped to bring about democratisation in Malawi, where the national bishops' pastoral letter of 1992, 'Living Our Faith', distributed to parishes across the country, was the first public criticism levelled against the one-party rule of Hastings Kamuzu Banda, and a turning point in bringing him down. Opposing post-colonial authoritarian regimes, the Church helped bring about democracy because of its political ideology of human rights and democracy. Philpott (2004) shows how the Catholic Church in Malawi spoke out against human rights abuses and poor governance in 1992. The church is therefore seen by local people as an important and positive force for change, making the views of its leadership highly influential.

Next, I show how the elites in Malawi churches have a key role in portraying cultural practices as negative and blaming them for the spread of HIV. The church has been key in distorting the impact sexual cultural practices have, linking them directly to AIDS.

The NGO Tearfund, a UK Christian relief and development agency, funded a meeting organised by the Evangelical Association of Malawi to 'use pastors to influence behaviour change and put a stop to cultural practices such as *kulowa kufa, fisi* and *kuchotsa fumbi*'; the practices to which I refer throughout this study. Here we see an oversimplification in the analysis of the link between cultural practices and AIDS. The article reports that abstinence and faithfulness among married couples will stop the spread of HIV, which contrasts with the article's conclusion, and the argument that cultural practices need to be stopped; however, the cultural practices listed do not involve married couples.

The following is an extract from an interview with PS the Member of Parliament who talks at length about the role of Christianity versus tradition:

> Aah, we aah, have been looking at the negative aspect of the cultural practices, and the government, the church, aah everybody international aah always writing about what is negative. (P5)

> He talks about a particular dance which is part of the initiation ceremony for the *fisi* practice said to spread HIV and he says "this great dance has caused a lot of problems to the early missionaries because they didn't understand it, but it has persisted, it has never been broken and over 150 years it is continuing". (P5)

This is an example of how the missionaries have not been able to change the culture. He goes on:

> From the Christian leaders aaah, it's a hangover from the early missionary perception that traditional customs are unchristian and in order to become a Christian, you had to renounce your membership or your practice of these... actually non-Christians are called *akunja, akunja* meaning outsiders, those who are outside the grace of God, whatever it is, as if God only created a certain people (laughter). Aaaah, when you do see one, aah, like try at the very first meeting to, to, to make, put your fact clearly that you are looking at it sympathetically, you respect what they ... whatever they will tell you, and if it is a secret and you don't want it to be defiled, I will respect it or whatever. Aaah then they will tell you a little bit more. But I have to be quite frank with you, you are not a chewa, they will never tell you everything, but at least enough for you to see the logic, aah and see why certain things are done in certain ways.
>
> I am quite radical about it ... we cannot allow this to happen, if our girls die, what will happen to the community, they were very concerned. But if several times you bombard them with 'change your habits' this is not good, a chief is a chief, miyambo he is the custodian of (laughs) this is undermining his own power. They will, they will respect you because it is the government, but you have not won their hearts. Aaah, where we, one of the objectives is to try to explain the Chewa customs, traditions, religion, art, culture, aaah dances to other Chewas as well as to other people. And we have, we hope that eventually we can have a radio station so that we can have our discussions freely without looking over our shoulders see whether our donors like it or not.
>
> But there is a lot of misunderstanding, a lot of ignorance, a lot of very early condemnation of the issues by people who don't understand, who don't know anything. Lastly, I wanted to, I mentioned that there would be some issues of the positives, in this short paper it is not published, but it's just some of my thinking. I, I, from what I have told you about the responsibility to the community, that is very positive, very powerful for our concern, and therefore, following on to that, there are institutions with traditional, traditional institutions which have been set up which we can utilize, I mentioned may be one or two, I mentioned one, it is here. It is here. One is the marriage counsellors, when the family starts, the woman has, has a *nkhoswe* as her counsellor, her sponsor so to speak. For a life time. The man also has his, these are the people who were there in the marriage negotiations. They start right at the beginning and if there are any problems, the family wants to discuss they call on these two people, one or two of these people. Now that's an institution which is almost,

which is only working now at the actual wedding. When the wedding is there, they say who is the *nkhoswe*, when they go in church they say who is the *nkhoswe*, who is the *nkhoswe* for this woman, who dadadada! That's the end. But that is the institutions traditionally which was there to for the young couple to confide, to discuss issues, if there are any problems they would come, that's one. The other, institution is the traditional court, the chief, the *bwalo* where the elders meet regularly. Aah elders means both male and female in the Chewa although they sit separately. But they go to the *bwalo* under the big tree, that also is a consultative forum and many issues are discussed every case, legal case that is that comes there it is resolved at the *bwalo* where the chief sits with his counsellors as judges. So that *bwalo* system can be used. Then the initiation structures themselves, are very powerful educational and training institutions. You know what the boys and girls learn during initiation stays with them the rest of their lives, they never forget them.

And as an educationist myself, I was interested to know how do they teach (laughter) these boys and girls that they don't forget? Yaah, its songs, proverbs, aaa ee sayings, similes. Our cultures are very symbolic. So the explanation of symbols and what it means aah through songs, but also the instruction is almost one to one. And the demonstration, the physical demonstrations are very important. They will tell you the theories et cetera, but then they demonstrate by some act may be if you are talking about death, you would think that they have brought a dead person there, but actually he is not dead, but the way they present (laughter), the young people get the message that you know, it's not something that is light, it has to be respected because the spirit has left the body yes, but it's there. It is another form of existence. So it is very much interesting. I haven't done much work there but it's amazing that they have been very successful in putting ... and then there is the issue of personal training as well because, if it is a girl, they are taught how to cook, how to look after the children, hygiene, how to look after the house, and this is very important.

Secondly, a Christian influence has been deeply assumed that what is Christian is good, and what a Christian says is bad is bad. And many people of our group have become Christians, have grown up like Christians and really even the Chewa, many Chewas that I talk to, don't know about their culture, they are surprised when I give them some lectures on Chewas religion was all about, and they say, but aaah Chewa religion is good (laughter). So the whole history of cultural suppression had its toll and really even in the west when this disease came, they really didn't know how to tackle it. So really nobody had experience. I would really want to jump to the easy explanation and yaah you are supposed to be curious object of the study, and so aaah, I think that's why I said, I think we missed a point in tackling HIV/AIDS. We would have done a better job. We would have done a better job if we went to the chief, to the namkungwi, and explained and had a dialogue with them and told, no one wants their child dead. I am sure that we would have found a very good solution. My wife used to work for UNICEF. (P5)

Despite him explaining about the influence of Christianity, he also makes it known to me that he is a member of the elite. He says as an educationist myself and then talks about his wife who used to work for UNICEF. By associating himself with his wife's position in a UN agency makes him an elite. Furthermore, as pointed out in the previous chapter, elites distance themselves from those communities that observe cultural practices and position themselves in opposition to them as more enlightened— defined as a reflection of ATR and conversion to Christianity.

The following is an extract from an interview with a journalist. I read an article in a national newspaper about cultural practices and AIDS. I emailed him and we agreed to meet at a radio station in Lilongwe. It was only upon arrival when I signed in I learnt that he was a Reverend and that the radio station was Christian. The radio station's mission is to assist the Church to fulfil the command of Jesus Christ to make disciples of all peoples, and to do so by using and making available mass media to proclaim the gospel of salvation to as many people as possible and instruct believers in biblical doctrine and daily Christ-like living. He told me that during the period of sixteen days against gender-based violence, he normally carries out some write-ups focusing on specific areas on the theme that is being set aside that year. I said to him that in his newspaper article he talks about cultural practices. I asked him if he honestly thinks the practices mentioned in his article contribute to the transmission of HIV. He responded:

> I think they do because if you look at most of the cultural practices of our concern those cultural practices that either have a stature component or have a component where you know some grievous bodily harm has to be inflicted in order to invoke the power of that particular practice. I mean if you look at *fisi* for instance I mean, its aah surrounding the question of infertility and so in order to resolve that infertility such sexual practice must happen. *Chokolo*, which is wife inheritance, it's the same thing there has to be some sexual activity between the lady and the relation of the dead man, aa same thing with *kulowa kufa*, you find that again it involves ritual sex and so on. Aaah, actually I just pulled a document from

my computer in which we will also see oppression, I think three years ago I attended a faith based leaders conference which was looking at some cultural practices which are fuelling the spread of HIV/AIDS in Malawi. I think this does look at quite a number of areas. If you look at these two the central slide which talk about sexual intercourse as ritual cleansing, sexual cleansing, cleansing a child initiation cleansing so you find that you know the sexual act has quite a very central role in aa in the cultural cleansing process. So aah one, one can't wish away these, one can't trivialize the role of you know, of sexual practices in our cultural practices. If you look at the last line there, sex as a coping mechanism and then where it says *Mwamuna ndi kabudula amathera moyenda, mwamuna sauzidwa*, it kind of justifies the fact that its natural for men to be promiscuous. But the husband, the man uses his common sense and common sense for him his wife alone is not sufficient. How loaded that particular statement *mamuna sauzidwa* may be. If you go to page three, there are 6 coping mechanisms. These are some of the practices one of them that I would like to talk about is *chisuweni*, the fourth one. *Nsuweni* means that if I have a cousin, *Msuweni* literally means cousin culturally there is freedom that you can flirt around because your cousin is not your sister and so there is that kind of social closeness between somebody and their cousins so you find that sexually it becomes very easy for people to sexually relate with their cousins. And then of course *Mitala* is polygamy, aaah, polygamy has got a role in the HIV/AIDS. The other talks about sex as a sign of hospitality, and, aah where you pay a visit to a village and then they give you a lady to actually entertain you over the night. So that's aaah the actual basis of some of those. *Kusamala mlendo* means taking care of visitors aah *nkhosa amamwa mkaka wa mberere zake...* to say that aah...... okay let me talk about the one which says *wamkachise amadya za mkachisi*. Its got some kind of religious connotation to say that if somebody is working in a temple, he has to eat, he has to take their livelihood within the temple which they are working in and that sometimes is used culturally to say that for instance if I am the chief of the village then I can have access to any woman that I want to have access to, aaah and so on and so forth. So this does outline some of those that are quite central in our cultural set up. (P3)

He said that the conference he attended was organised by the Norwegian Church Aid where church leaders were brought together to speak about gender-based violence. I explained that the probability of the girl becoming infected in one sexual act with a fisii is one in one thousand. He said: 'For the young virgin'. I said: 'Well for anyone. And if the person has a sexually transmitted infection, then the probability of catching the virus... is every eight in one thousand'. He said: 'Oh! when

5 HOW THE CHURCH FRAMES AIDS   119

you talk about that statistics you are talking about, for me it's the first time as well to encounter that' (P3). This point demonstrates how he was unaware of the disease's epidemiology. It is also an example of how the church is able to powerfully communicate its message through the media. He then went on to say:

> Yaah its clear that those types of messages have come up through quite well, I think the impression created in one way aaah aaah, every sexual encounter, potentially, yah potentially you know, can infect you with the virus. But then, aaa I think the issue is one where we do not want to say ... the messages stem from a technical point of view that if viewed from the information and the moment the public gets the information, aaaaah the public are already threatened then they ... that defeats the whole process of behaviour change ....But to answer your question, it's a, in that scenario of aaah initiation, its chances are that aaah, from just a single sexual act, that doesn't transmit the virus. Perhaps that then calls for a longitudinal research aaah we need the information in Malawi so that we would be able to determine all these claims we are meeting regarding cultural practices that are fuelling the spread of AIDS. If eeeh aaah, can we make evidence based claims. (P3)

In his response, he justifies why he did not know about the disease's probability of infection by arguing that it is better not to tell the public the truth about the disease, otherwise this defeats the process of behaviour change. In other words, he is making points: (i) don't tell the public the truth about the disease and (ii) people will not change their behaviour if they know that the probability of infection is so low. In the quote above, the respondent seems to be patronising the 'other' as he refers to the public as separate from himself and defines them as uneducated. He then went on to talk about the sexualisation of women:

> One does see those types of linkages. Aaah some of it is aah in terms of some of the cultural practices, I think, whether they fuel HIV, the spread of HIV/AIDS, personally I think that its very clear that the very practice of them does usually subject a woman to inhumane treatment where the woman is treated more of as a sexual object as opposed to the fact that they should govern their own wellbeing. The observation that is being made in most forums that I have attended is that because we have been too quick to condemn cultural practices, you find that where we are celebrating that they are not being eradicated, they are simply going into hiding. (P3)

I interviewed a District Youth Officer who previously worked as a field facilitator for a faith-based organisation called Family Life and AIDS Education Ministry that trained community volunteers on AIDS based on biblical principles. He said:

> people have to understand that HIV cancellation is through spiritual conduct, if they avoid that they are going to prevent from contracting the virus and for them to do that they have to understand that God hates immorality. (P15)

He said that he does not belong to any church as its interdenominational funded by Oikomonos Foundation from the Netherlands (the Oikonomos foundation is a Christian organisation working on development cooperation and works with local partner organisations in Bolivia, Ghana, Indonesia, India, Malawi, Nigeria and Zimbabawe)—a further example of international donors funding religious activities. He said:

> We were teaching them that at least as a family, if they enjoy the family life they have to follow the big responsibility, God instituted the family so that the two, the husband and the wife should live happily, what is happening is that the two are not living happily because they have ignored what God has instituted, so we are trying to teach them that, and again if they had heard to what the Bible said about family life, they are also going to avoid contracting the virus that causes AIDS. (P15)

He then went on to explain about cultural practices:

> R: There are a lot of cultural practices that are being practiced in Mulanje and Thyolo where we have been working, so we are tackling that like *kuchosa fumbi*, *chokolo*, how many do you want? *kulowa fisi*... yeah there are many of them.
> S: But what are you doing about these practices?
> R: For example this *kuchosa fumbi* is practiced during initiation ceremonies, for example after initiation ceremonies they are advised to shake off their dust that is they should have sex. So sometimes we could go to where the initiation ceremonies were taking place and we could advise them that they should stop because it promotes the spread of HIV/AIDS. And again we could go to churches because some of these people who were involved in initiation ceremonies, the *anankungwi*

initiation councilors were coming from the churches, so we could go through the churches and talk to them and say look at what the word of God is saying, advise them on this, and not only that, we could also advise the councilors that if they want to cut the foreskin, they should not use the same razor blade, at least each young man should have his razor blade so that they should avoid contracting the virus that causes HIV/AIDS.

He went on to explain that he trained volunteers from the surrounding communities about cultural practices so 'they could go and teach others'. In return:

As a token of appreciation, I don't know what I can call this, they could receive something like we were giving them bicycles which they were using to have their ceremonies in the communities and not only that, sometimes we could give them some soap, flour, salt, fertilizer, maize seeds, not as a payment for the work they were doing but....

I asked about the training that takes place:

S: Okay, do cultural practices come up?
R: Yeah it comes out automatically, we have a lesson on that and some of the cultural practices that I have mentioned come out automatically
S: Why?
R: Some of them are being practiced here in Balaka, so when we take the young men and women for training, we ask them to give some cultural practices that are practiced in their respective areas and what they say it's what I have already said about Thyolo and Mulanje.
S: So what do you teach them about?
R: Cultural practices, firstly they have to understand what the cultural practices are all about and why are they practiced. This comes in the course of the discussion as a facilitator and the participant.
S: Say for example, I am a participator, what do you tell me about cultural practices?
R: I ask you what cultural practices are being practiced from where you are coming from, so you mention them, maybe you brainstorm about them and then you start to discuss are these good?, if they are bad, how are they bad?
S: So what do they say are good?
R: Of course there are some cultural practices that are good, not all are bad, but for those that are bad like the *Kusasa fumbi*, that one is very

dangerous because it promotes the spread of HIV/AIDS, after the initiation ceremonies, they are told to have sex with the male youth or female youth and in the course of having sex may be the female youth has the virus, she is going to spread that virus to the male youth and if the male youth has the virus, he is going to spread that virus to the female youth.

S: So let's think about it, you say to young people, what are you trying to advise when they are having sex?

R: Yeah, if they might not have sex before, they might not spread the virus, but it's not only the issue of HIV/AIDs, there are issues like pregnancy, they can impregnate and on the STIs, we don't talk about HIV/AIDS alone, there are some infections like gonorrhoea, syphilis and others so we discuss about the dangers of such things. If you contract the virus that causes HIV/AIDS at one time or the other you will suffer from AIDS and it will jeopardize your health and as a result of this the future is doomed.

S: And that's the Ministry of Health (MoH) incorporating cultural practices in your training, what, where do they come from?

R: It's not the issues of incorporating they were already there.

S: You have talked about cultural practices, so is it already incorporated in your training manual or...

R: Yes it's already in our training manual, we have it and you can see it.

Here we see that although he mentions 'good' and 'bad' cultural practices he only tells me about the bad ones that those are very 'dangerous'. It is interesting that the Malawians themselves make the practices exotic as if I will be impressed to hear about them. We go on to talk about geographical areas where the training is conducted.

S: Do you go to all areas?

R: Yeah we go to all areas and there are youth groups in all areas. There are some areas where cultural practices are being practiced more than other areas like the areas where there are Yaos, this Kalembo side, Kachinga side, Amidu side and part of Nsamala.

S: Predominantly it's among the Yao?

R: Yes! Amongst the Yao.

S: But other tribes do it too?

R: Other tribes, off course they do it but not as the Yao do it.

S: What do you mean?

R: Yaos are doing it much much greater than the other tribes because the other tribes are mixing with other tribes, they have tried to reduce it, but these Yao people, they are difficult to change.

S: Why do you think it's that?

R: I do not know, may be because of the way they were brought up or we just established that these are very difficult to change and we have to follow that, this is what our ancestors, our father were doing so we have to do it. The other thing is that, these people they have problems with school, they do not go to school, you know education also influences once you know to change behaviour so amongst the Yao, you cannot find many people who have gone to school, you will find a 12, or 14 year old female youth is married and is carrying a baby on her back, why.. because of the cultural practices, if you tell them about school, they don't feel the need for them to go to school, maybe because of a lack of role models among themselves, there are no role models, they haven't seen somebody who has gone to school who has completed his or her studies and is working or doing fine because of school, for example, myself, I went to school and I am now working, if I was coming from a Yao area they could emulate my example that he is doing fine because he went to school, so such role models are not present amongst the Yaos. Those that could become role models are no longer there, they left a long time ago and they cannot go back to their respective areas to influence their relatives that you people this is what you are supposed to be doing, so you go to them, you tell them about the badness of those cultural practices but because there are no role models amongst themselves, it becomes difficult for them to change. And somebody amongst the Yaos said that, if you are coming here for your lessons, make sure that you are coming with a sharp axe.

S: Why?

R: They said that not many of us Yaos have gone to school so for us to understand some of the things you are talking about it becomes very difficult, so come with a sharp axe and cut all the roots so that we can change our behaviour, so there are a lot of work amongst the Yao.

S: What does the government do to try to make them to go to school?

R: There a lot of schools, they just start from standard one to standard five then they drop and get married.

S: How old do they reach standard five?

R: About eleven or twelve. So those that are doing fine among the Yaos, for example I am from Blantyre and I am working as a teacher I go and settle there, my children are also learning there they are the ones that are doing fine in their studies not the Yaos themselves. (P15)

This interview extract shows how he is portraying himself as an elite and in this case he is blaming the Yao tribe.

One woman worked for the Evangelical Association of Malawi (EAM). She explained:

> It's an umbrella organisation of TransWorld Radio, Pentecostal and Evangelical Churches, now almost 82 churches and organisations. The Christian Health Association of Malawi is affiliated, EAM is its umbrella. Its core purpose is preaching the gospel but then it realized that there's a need for social services. HIV/AIDS is just one of the projects, with funding from DanChurch.
>
> When beginning a project we normally conduct research, so we did that in about five districts. We learned about cultural practices, normally known as the *fisi*. *Fisi* for families that don't have children is common in the central region and in the south. Then we have the *fisi* in the Central region for ritual cleansing for girls reaching puberty, the parents look for a man to cleanse her, the girl is supposed to do that just because it's culture. And have it for ritual cleansing, especially in the south, when the husband has died. (P55)

I asked 'What do you do to try to change the cultural practices that are a perceived to be a problem?' She said 'We mobilize the traditional leaders, headmen. For the church it's not difficult, our teaching is based on the Bible, in the Bible we have to wait until we get married to have sex. But for traditional leaders who are the custodians of the culture, we normally conduct trainings'. I asked what do you tell them in the trainings?

> The definition of AIDS, how it is spread, which cultural practices spread it. If possible we encourage their wives to attend. If it's a she we encourage the husband to attend. We tell them how they can prevent infection, or if they are infected how they can prevent transmission. We tell them, the parents, that you take a man [for a *fisi*] but you don't have him tested, you don't know what he is. And then the girl gets married. But not to the *fisi* he is just gone. (P55)

> Before the training ends we develop an action plan, that helps us in monitoring. If they are really doing what they wrote on their action plan'. Normally they say at the end of the training we didn't know this but now that we know we are going to sensitize our community in an awareness campaign, we are going to involve the youths so there can be some songs on HIV/AIDS, so there can be dramas. It is easy to engage the youth'. (P55)

She said the practices are immoral and that most of the communities where missionaries first came they were the first to stop them. She said that AIDS and cultural practices are parallel issues. 'For us social workers we would love to identify the issues in whatever we are doing'. Then she talks about stigma in the church, that people who have AIDS are called sinners, 'the church would say everyone who has the virus is a sinner. But EAM doesn't want to say this, we don't want to say *fisii* are immoral. We started working on AIDS prevention in 1999 and cultural practices in 2003 because as we were working with the religious leaders, issue of stigma came out. But the community was finding it difficult to accommodate those with the virus in the communities'. Then there were talks about hunger; that they give out maize. 'That helped create stigma, since they had to identify as HIV positive to get the maize'. This started to fight stigma. That's when we started to approach the traditional leaders because they were stigmatising, so they said you traditional leaders are also at fault you are spreading HIV. The question was posed 'I would think they wouldn't want you to come to their village?' 'No No', she said. We were going there humbly [she clasped her hands and looked down, respectfully]. We would first meet the religious leaders, and then they would meet with the chiefs' (P55).

Two people I interviewed showed me the same presentation that was given by the Evangelical Association of Malawi at regional and national church leaders' meetings. The presentation depicts 20 slides; the first one entitled 'Evangelical Association of Malawi—Cultural Practices'. The second slide poses the question—what is fuelling the spread of HIV infection in Malawi? One slide then shows the factors that increase community vulnerability to HIV/AIDS and includes cultural and religious practices and lack of biblical sound teaching. The presentation goes on to identify different types of sexual acts which purportedly spread HIV including sexual intercourse for cleansing, sex as a coping mechanism, sex as a factor for hospitality, sex as a factor of entertainment and sex as a treatment or cause of problem (i.e. health problems from not having sex and sex causing cancer).

I interviewed the Coordinator for HIV/AIDS, Nutrition and Health at World Vision, Balaka. She is a qualified nurse. She explained 'We do advocacy. We also work hand in hand with community leaders, the chiefs, church leaders and faith leaders. Sometimes we just hold a discussion with community leaders on cultural practices in the area and how that, those cultural practices contribute to HIV/AIDS. Sometimes we engage drama groups to come and just entertain people. We are educating people about the disadvantages of those cultural practices'. I asked if she found that community leaders are willing to change the practices? She said 'You just notice the change in behaviour. What they say. Issues of stigma and discrimination. They wouldn't mix with those people with HIV/AIDS. They would not talk openly. They are freely talking about it now. Normally talking about sexual practices is taboo'. I asked if she had heard the community leaders talking? Firstly she said Yes. I said Are they saying they have changed them? She said No you actually notice them talking. A chief would say something encouraging. I said why do you think that? She said the reason I am saying it is I have actually seen community leaders talking about it (P42).

The above extract is peppered with development buzzwords—'advocacy, stigma and discrimination, change in behaviour'. Buzzwords are, what Williams (1976) called 'keywords': words that evoke, and come to carry, the cultural and political values of the time. Such words are frequently used in the language of mainstream development but it is often unclear what these words actually mean and what they do for development policy. It is therefore significant because the woman is using these words without referencing the meaning behind them. She is demonstrating the use of development policy language but gives no concrete examples evidencing how behaviour change has actually taken place.

The Malawi Interfaith AIDS Association (MIAA) submitted a proposal to UNFPA entitled 'Combating HIV/AIDS through Elimination of Cultural and Religious Practices' and aligned its objectives with those of UNFPA. This is an example of how national organisations adopt the language of international donors to secure funding. In MIAA's proposal, it stated:

> Faith-based institutions and organisations could have a profound impact on the HIV/AIDS pandemic when they are properly and adequately equipped with the right skills and knowledge to facilitate their work. Religious institutions as trusted and respected institutions are better placed to play a significant role in the fight against HIV/AIDS. Faith-based institutions can effectively encourage and support loving, just and honest relationships and encourage members of the faith communities to adopt behaviours that renounce and repulse any traits of gender inequality, cultural and religious practice as well as stigma and discrimination that exacerbate HIV transmission by using religious and spiritual teachings in a positive way while at the same time offer compassion and promote

reconciliation. Many Malawians (over 95 percent) belong to most of the faith institutions in the country.

Despite the realization of this critical role that the faith-based institutions could play in the fight against the epidemic, most religious and traditional leaders still do not have the requisite knowledge and skills to wage the war. MIAA Secretariat is requesting financial support from UNFPA intends to strengthen the capacities of the religious and traditional leaders who are the custodian of culture and the congregants to effectively respond to the pandemic. It is expected that through this support faith and traditional leaders and the congregants themselves will cultivate amongst their congregants positive behaviours that also contribute to an effective fight against gender inequality and cultural and religious practices that facilitate HIV transmission.

Using data from desk research and culturally sensitive approaches, the proposed project seeks to conduct some training programmes, social mobilization and advocacy sessions for both religious and traditional leaders and the congregants with the view of building their capacity to play an active and positive role in the fight against gender inequality, cultural and religious practice as well as stigma and discrimination. (n.d., MIAA funding proposal)

MIAA told me that they intended to design a programme called Mpaka Liti. The programme would fight against gender inequalities and social injustices that are deeply rooted in the cultural and religious norms and tradition in Malawi. In this programme, communities and religious institutions will be challenged to realise that it was about time that things needed to change for the better. In addition, the leaders will spearhead a campaign to modify or completely eliminate the major cultural, religious and traditional practices that are driving the HIV transmission in the country. They would also:

'Conduct training sessions for members of District Interfaith AIDS Committees in basic facts about the theology of HIV/AIDS. This will help to strengthen the capacity of the traditional and religious leaders to assess and analyse their own personal narratives in relation to the intersections between violence and HIV/AIDS) and conduct training sessions for religious leaders and other influential people within the faith institution'. (P52)

The respondent working for World Vision in Balaka told me when I asked: 'Do you talk about cultural practices and HIV/AIDS?' She said:

There are many. We have a practice that we call *fisi* – where like I am married and my husband is dead then to drive the evil spirits away I have to sleep with another man. Then there is this belief that for you to be recognised as a man in the society you have to have multiple sexual partners. The other one is..ok..something is… If I am HIV+when you sleep with an albino the HIV will go away. Yah *Kusasa fumbi* - It's the same as *fisi*. It's where..and some of the beliefs or rather the cultures is like, yah, when I reach puberty, yah, I have to sleep with a man for me to be recognised as a woman. I ask 'Is that part of the chinamwali?' Yes it's chinamwali. When you reach puberty they take you away for some counselling and the like. And at the end they give you a man to sleep with. (P42)

As demonstrated in this chapter in an attempt to change people's behaviours, respondents repeatedly asserted that religious leaders need to be targeted. The following excerpt has been taken from a leaflet I was given when I visited MANERELA+'s office which is a further example of educating religious leaders.

MANARELA+ Leaflet Excerpt
MANERELA+ Malawi Network of Religious Leaders Living with or Personally Affected by AIDS

Launched in 2004 by Reverend Canon Gideon Byamugisha. Purpose of MANERELA+ is to prevent and mitigate the impact of HIV/AIDS through the reduction of Stigma, Silence, Denial, Discrimination, Inaction and Misaction (SSDIM) at community and national level.

Specific objectives:
To promote safer and lawful sexual practices and behaviours through the SAVE model.

To improve networking and collaboration among the religious leaders living with or personally affected by HIV/AIDS and the key stakeholders.

The network works hand in hand with stakeholders and other institutions such as MANASO, MANET+, NAPHAM, MIAA, EAM, NAC, Action Aid, Ecumenical Counselling Centre, District interfaith AIDS Committee (DIAC), World Vision International, MAM.

Strategies. The network will fight SSDIM through advocacy, media theological debates or forums, training the religious leaders and other people living with HIV, adherence and peer counsellors training, national retreats, capacity building of the network, gender and human rights mainstreaming and promotion of networking and collaboration, development and distribution of relevant information, education and communication, materials and establishment of district and regional clusters of group therapy.

Working in Mzimba, Mzuzu, Salima, Mwanza, Dedza, Nkhotakota, Machinga and Mulanje. Funding partners: Norwegian Church Aid; The Southern African AIDS Trust and Christian Aid.

I interviewed a Programme Officer working for the Norwegian Church Aid. She has a Master's degree and wrote her thesis on religious leaders and AIDS. When I first arrived in her office, she gave me a copy of the study that the Evangelical Association of Malawi carried out on cultural and religious beliefs and practices. This was the same study the Reverend gave me when I interviewed him at the radio station. It is interesting that out of 3 interviews, three interviewees shared with me that same study. She told me Norwegian Church Aid works on a number of areas on HIV/AIDS. It is working with two partners focusing on HIV/AIDS in the Lower Shire, specifically Chikwawa and Nsanje. In Nsanje they are working with the Episcopal Conference of Malawi and the Chikwawa Health Commission, as she said: 'cultural practices are prevalent there in Chikwawa', so they are disseminating information on 'sensitisation and awareness'. I asked what do they actually do in terms of sensitisation and awareness? She said: 'The Chikwawa Health Commission produces IEC materials like T-Shirts which say on the front 'Let us stop harmful cultural practices'. It works with the Catholic Commission for Justice and Peace through media programmes on the radio as well as trying to emphasise restricting cleansing rites such as *Chokolo*'. Here we see the use of development buzzwords once again: sensitisation and awareness. When I probe her, she responds with 'IEC'. In fact she assumes I understand what IEC means as she uses the acronym. By using these words she is demonstrating that she is educated and familiar with development policy. Coupled by her fluency in which she uses this language, and that she is a Programme Officer working for an international NGO based in the capital, she can be described as a member of the Malawian national elite (P56).

I asked her if she thought these cultural practices contribute to the spread of AIDS? 'Yes in my opinion the effects spread HIV. Young boys and girls get infected. The man who sleeps with the girls, he slept with more than one girl. He sleeps with all girls'. I asked how are the boys infected? 'Circumcision. One razor blade is used. And also how to do sex with a woman after initiation'. She said if we look at prevalence rates, 1 in 10 people are being infected. She also said 'If we look at specific activities one of the areas being identified is harmful cultural practices. The evidence is the predisposing area' (P56).

Her other argument was that if you take groups of people living with AIDS, one man said that he was the man who had to have sex with young girls and that is how he became infected. This argument doesn't actually weigh up since the man would be having sex with virgins and therefore would not get infected by the virgins. She said that again we need to look at statistics and existing documentation. She said that in urban areas we have antenatal clinics so there are more statistics for urban areas. I said that in rural areas we also have the Behavioural Sentinel Surveillance data. She then argued that people from rural areas come to urban areas so that is how the disease is being spread around and that those from rural areas are bringing it to the urban areas. This is a further example of blaming the rural villager who visits urban areas and then spreads the disease to the elites. She said it is not just an issue of having sex but people having access to information. Information, she argued, is not available. We know this is not true as evidence shows that Malawians are aware of AIDS. She also says 'It is also an issue of poverty. In our culture people are being encouraged to get married early – this is a cultural practice'. She also talked about the issue of being sick where the same razor blade is used and this contributes to AIDS. What she says here shows how she is confusing many issues and is not clear how much of the actual epidemiology of AIDS she is aware of.

Interestingly, one respondent stated:

> About the religious groups, they are making progress but the most difficult are the Pentecostal and evangelical group. (P5)

This next section looks at the role of religion and sexual cultural practices to understand why they are still observed despite the increased accessibility of biomedicine and education. The reason why I am addressing this issue is to support my argument—why are the cultural practices being observed—but also the way in which the church is trying to distance itself from the practices therefore presenting itself as more enlightened.

Research conducted by van Gennep (1960) and subsequently Turner suggest that the meaning and significance of religion is entrenched and transmitted through rituals. For Turner (1967), 'ritual' applies to forms of religious behaviour associated with social transitions. According to Longwe (2007), initiation rites form an integral part of contemporary

Chewa culture. She argues that apart from the sociological and cultural importance, it is within the religious context that initiation rites have the most significant impact on Chewa society. Oduyoye (1992) holds the view that African rituals are psychological, spiritual, political and social. According to Turner (1967), the term 'ceremony' has a closer bearing on religious behaviour associated with social states, where politico-legal institutions also have greater importance. Ritual is described as transformative, ceremony as confirmatory.

Initiation ceremonies are often used for sex education because in Malawi the mother is not allowed to talk about sex to her daughter. Mbugua (2007) highlights this using data from a study conducted in 1996 and 2003 which examines the sociocultural and religious factors that prevent educated mothers in urban Kenya from teaching sex-education to their pre-adolescent and adolescent daughters. She concluded that sociocultural and religious inhibitions prevent educated mothers in urban Kenya from giving meaningful sex-education to their pre-adolescent and adolescent daughters.

I now quote extensively from Longwe's book *Growing Up – A Chewa Girls' Initiation* to give context on why a girl experiences initiation:

> When a girl experiences her first menstruation she undergoes a ceremony called *chikule* performed for a smooth transition from childhood to adulthood. The belief among the Chewa is that menstrual blood is sacred and that it has mysterious powers of sustaining human life. Proper rituals must be performed and all taboos observed so that nothing endangers her life and that of the whole community so that she should not become sterile or suffer *mdulo*. Whoever notices the girl's first menses must inform the mother immediately who in turn informs the grandmother. The chief, as the owner of the *mbumba* and the one responsible for the girl's initiation, is also informed through his *anankungwi* (instructresses).
>
> The taboos to be observed during the girl's first menstruation are sexual abstinence for the parents until the end of her menses when the rituals described below are performed. The chief abstains only in the case of a girl who will be initiated at *mkangali* (the chief's initiation, as discussed below). All informants mentioned that if the parents break the sexual taboo the girl suffers from a disease called *mdulo* or *tsempho*. The symptoms of *mdulo* or *tsempho* are *kutupa masaya, kusololoka zala, kusanza magazi* or *kutuwa* (swollen cheeks, elongated fingers, vomiting blood or rough dry skin) and eventually the girl dies if not given the necessary herbs to cure the illness. In normal circumstances the girl is given food without

salt and is instructed not to salt any food whenever she is menstruating. The grandmother's role is to take the girl into two or three days seclusion for instruction concerning her menses. The girl is warned of the dangers of having sex during menstruation, and she is instructed on how to take care of the menses so that no one sees the blood, nor the menses linen, called *mwele* or *mthete*. She is instructed to respect her parents, the elderly people and especially the chief. At the end of her menses, the chief provided the necessary herbal medicine, called *khundabwi*, for the girl to eat in food or to drink with the parents (and the grandmother). Again the chief eats *khundabwi* only in the case of the special girl who will undergo mkangali. After taking the herbal medicine, all are free to resume their sexual activity.

Many informants mentioned that in the past, instead of the herbal medicine the girl was given a man to have sex with at night. Such a man was called *fisi* (hyena) because he came at night as a 'hyena to steal'. The warning for both the girl and the man was as one informant stated 'this must be kept as a secret and that it was just a one time ritual not to be repeated or continued'. Some informants said that this practice was the cause of polygamous families, for some men decided to marry the girl after the ritual act. In some cases it was the cause for premarital pregnancies among girls for some men continued to meet with the girl secretly. However, few informants insisted that the ritual is still practiced in spite of the HIV/AIDS pandemic. Their argument is that the family looks for someone whom they see as HIV/AIDS free, for they claim that the elderly women, just by looking someone in the eyes, are able to identify those who are sick. (Longwe 2007, pp. 41–42)

Fisi may be given to a girl to purify her at the end of her first menses. In this case she is tested for pregnancy and not sexual purity (p. 60). However most of the instruction is to 'please' the husband (p. 65). Phiri argued that the importance of female initiation rites is demonstrated by the Chewa, who have four initiation ceremonies for women.

Christian's Response to the Chinamwali

Research conducted by Turner (1967) and van Gennep (1960) suggest that the meaning and significance of religion is entrenched and transmitted through rituals. According to Longwe (2007), initiation rites form an integral part of contemporary Chewa culture. Longwe argues that apart from the sociological and cultural importance, it is within the religious context that initiation rites have most significant impact on Chewa society. *Fisi* may be given to a girl to purify her at the end of her first menses. In this case she is tested for pregnancy and not sexual purity (p. 60). Phiri argued that the importance of female initiation rites is demonstrated by the Chewa who have four initiation ceremonies for women and that most of the instruction is to 'please' the husband (p. 65). Longwe also talks about meetings with the Baptist church and a group of Malawian leaders talk about a national committee which had meetings to discuss a book that the Church wanted to write. The main argument was on their differences in some traditional customs, especially between rural and urban women (p. 78). Furthermore, female church members reported difficulties with what the church was saying, telling them that practices surrounding the life cycle rituals were unchristian and breaking away from some of these practices for fear of the consequences (p. 102). Sexual purity is not taught in traditional chewa society since girls can be introduced to sex on their first menses (p. 113).

In a document produced by the Evangelical Association of Malawi (EAM) entitled *EAM HIV/AIDS Programme: Baseline Survey Report*, 28 cultural practices were listed which purportedly spread HIV/AIDS, including the *fisi* practice. In the report it stated that:

> The irony of these practices is that they are still being practiced with more than 84% record of Christianity, and where all the mainland churches have already had their centenary cerebrations of their existence. During the focus group discussions with members of the church, it sounded as if issues of sexual immorality and witchcraft are deeply rooted and imbedded in culture such that the Christian faith cannot get rid of it or have it changed. It sounded as like; the Christian faith is far from transforming a culture. As if to confirm this, during the focus group discussions, the church members were emphasising that these practices can not be changed and people can never stop doing these practices. At one group discussion women lamented that such type of immoral practices are just part of our living, and being given a man for sexual intercourse, whether the woman or girl likes it or not is something that we as women have to live with. As women, the women continued, we are hired a man who is sometimes extremely dirty and filthy to have sexual intercourse with, in which case we have to do it because that is what is expected of us, or else, from the woman's own initiative, we take the trouble of bathing and cleaning this man before having sexual intercourse with him. Members of the church are practicing these traditions to the extent that some of the hired men and women are leaders of the church at different positions. (EAM Report, n.d., p. 12)

This paragraph reveals the use of moralising language such as references to practices as 'immoral' or 'bad' without any attempt to clarify the cultural rationales for the rituals. Associated with this is the accusation that people are unwilling to 'change', and are portrayed as conservative and backward and that the church is unable to 'transform' the culture. It also reveals that women are powerless and are forced to have sex with men and cannot say no. Yet research suggests people are making several changes in their practices both everyday and 'cultural' as outlined in newspaper articles (Schatz 2005; Smith and Watkins 2005; Kalipeni and Ghosh 2007).

I interviewed a Community Development Officer working for Balaka District Assembly. He highlighted the importance of cultural issues in rural areas:

> Aah you know cultural issues are regarded as very very important behaviour in a village setting. Aaah as a district first of all our aim is to *enlighten the community* on these cultural issues because they have been with these cultural issues since time immemorial. (P14)

This comment demonstrates how he makes the link between cultural issues and rural areas, but also this comment has religious connotations using the word enlighten. It also is an example of educating the other: we need to enlighten them.

The church adopted three stages of traditional rites—puberty, marriage and pregnancy. The traditional instructresses (anankungwi) were replaced with the Christian instructresses. These Christian instructresses worked under the supervision and training of the women missionaries (Longwe 2007, p. 74). Missionaries adopted the initiation rites which were taught to the instructresses. It was compulsory for church members' children to attend the Christian initiation rite. The Christianised puberty rite included the instruction on the 'sanctity of the body and the respect due to it, physical implications of puberty, behaviour towards men and elders'. As Phiri pointed out in her observations on the initiation of Chewa women of Malawi:

> The public ceremony was held in the evening in a secluded 'well-lit' hall within the village, with all the initiates dressed in white. The programme for the evening was: opening prayer, singing of hymns, sharing of Word of

God, some instructions to the girls, welcoming the girls into the group of women by shaking hands, hymn and prayer. (Phiri 1998, p. 212)

Longwe also talks about meetings with the Baptist church and a group of Malawian leaders to discuss a book that the church wanted to write: 'the main argument was on their differences in some traditional customs, especially between rural and urban women' (Longwe 2007, p. 78). Furthermore, female church members reported difficulties with what the church was saying, telling them that practices surrounding the life-cycle rituals were unchristian and breaking away from some of these practices for fear of the consequences (p. 102). This point highlights the church's concern to distance itself from tradition positioning a more 'pure' form of Christianity as more enlightened. Sexual purity is not taught in traditional Chewa society since girls can be introduced to sex on their first menses (Longwe 2007, p. 113) and are required not to be pregnant during the time of chinamwali whether married or not. *Chinamwali* is not just about sex education but has a deeper religious meaning—establishing fertility for the initiates (p. 113). According to Longwe biblical teaching on good morals:

> Will help girls (and boys) to abstain from sex before marriage and to remain faithful during marriage. Jesus brings new life to the Chewa people. He gives added inward empowerment against sexual sin. Against this is a juxtaposition with tradition and trying to modernize a culture. The scriptures teach sexual purity until marriage and sexual faithfulness in marriage. Sexual purity also protects the girls from contracting the deadly disease of HIV/AIDS. (Longwe 2007, p. 113)

She believes that if instructresses consistently carry out Christian *chinamwali* and give continuous instruction to the girls, there should be no room for double initiations—secretly the traditional one first and later the church one: 'Let the initiates be taught how to live as adults and Christians in society' (p. 117).

One informant gave his opinion of the *chinamwali*:

> Aaah, because of this emphasis on fertility, aah now issues of sex through which they understood, is the way through which the children come, unlike there are some cultures in the pacific, they don't associate sex with reproduction (laughs), very funny (laughs), but Chewas looked at the

sexual act as part of the creation, reproduction, the continuation of God's power to increase humanity and so it is sacred, it has to be regulated by *miyambo*, its eeh, *miyambo* is translated as customs, but the word customs does not really capture the meaning of *miyambo*. *Miyambo* will also include ethical code in it, and not just a custom, a habit no, aah it's a code, and ethics around the responsibilities to the community. Every *mwambo*, *mwambo* is singular, is for the betterment of the individual, within the community so during this, in this are you have to have all these regulations to ensure that the community increases. (P6)

Conclusion

In this chapter, I demonstrated how Christian religious elites portray themselves as enlightened. They perceive cultural practices as harmful because they are practised primarily, perhaps only, in the rural areas by uneducated backward farmers—those who practise them are not modern. It is not clear whether harmful cultural practices became a priority in Malawi's HIV prevention policies at the beginning of the epidemic or only once NGOs began prioritising ending the epidemic by stopping these practices. Regardless of how the focus on cultural practices deemed to be harmful, it is interesting how the religious elites volunteer information on sexual cultural practices and enjoy talking about them. By referring to the sexual cultural practices at length, they distance themselves from the villagers who supposedly carry out these practices and conveniently apportion blame for HIV/AIDS away from them.

References

Barnett, T., & Parkhurst, J. (2005). HIV/AIDS: Sex, abstinence, and behaviour change. *The Lancet Infectious Diseases, 5*(9), 590–593.

Barrett, D. B., Kurian, G. T., & Johnson, T. M. (Eds.). (2001). *World Christian encyclopedia: A comparative survey of churches and religions in the modern world*. New York: Oxford University Press.

Bascom, W. R., & Herskovits, M. J. (1962). *Continuity and change in African cultures*. Chicago: University of Chicago Press.

Becker, F., & Geissler, P. W. (2007). Searching for pathways in a landscape of death: Religion and AIDS in East Africa. *Journal of Religion in Africa, 37*, 1–15.

Bratton, M. (1989). The politics of government-NGO relations in Africa. *World Development, 17*(4), 569–587.

Caldwell, J. C., Anarfi, J., Awusabo-Asare, K., Ntozi, J., Oruboloye, I. O., Marck, J., et al. (Eds.). (1999). *Resistances to behavioural change to reduce HIV/AIDS infection in predominantly heterosexual epidemics in third world countries*. Canberra: Australian National University.

Chaves, M. (2002). Religious organisations: Data resources and research opportunities. *American Behavioral Scientist, 45*(10), 1523–1549.

Evangelical Association of Malawi (EAM). (n.d.). *HIV/AIDS programme* (Baseline Survey Report). EAM, Blantyre.

Gallup News Service. (2007). *Africans' confidence in institutions—Which country stands out?* News Release. Retrieved October 20, 2013, from http://www.gallup.com/poll/26176/africans-confidence-institutions-which-country-stands-out.aspx.

Gama, H. (2000). Malawi churches brand condoms as immoral. *Africa News Service*, 5.

Gifford, P. (1998). *African Christianity: Its public role*. Bloomington: Indiana University Press.

Gifford, I. (2004). *Ghana's new Christianity: Pentecostalism in a globalising African economy*. London: Hurst & Company.

Gilmore, D. D. (1990). *Manhood in the making: Cultural concepts of masculinity*. New Haven and London: Yale University Press.

Harbeson, J., Rothchild, D., & Chazan, N. (Eds.). (1994). *Civil society and the state in Africa*. Boulder, CO: Lynne Rienner Publishers.

Jenkins P. (2007). *The next Christendom: The coming of global Christianity*. New York: Oxford University Press. http://www.amazon.com/Philip-Jenkins/e/B001IGLXQ0/ref=ntt_athr_dp_pel_1/176-3886970-8699844.

Jenkins, P. (2011). *The next Christendom: The coming of global Christianity*. OUP USA.

Kaler, A. (2004). AIDS-talk in everyday life: The presence of HIV/AIDS in men's informal conversation in Southern Malawi. *Social Science and Medicine, 59*(2), 285–297.

Kalipeni, E., & Ghosh, J. (2007). Concern and practice among men about HIV/AIDS in low socioeconomic areas of Lilongwe, Malawi. *Social Science and Medicine, 64*(5), 1116–1127.

Longwe, H. (2007). *Democratization of the Christian faith: The influence of the Baptist Doctrine of the "priesthood of all believers" on the history of the Baptist Convention of Malawi (BACOMA)*. University of Malawi.

Lwanda, J. (2005). *Politics, culture and medicine in Malawi*. Zomba: Kachere.

Mbiti, J. S. (1970). *Concepts of god in Africa*. London: SPCK.

Mbugua, N. (2007). Factors inhibiting educated mothers in Kenya from giving meaningful sex education to their daughters. *Social Science and Medicine, 64*(5), 1079–1089.

Oduyoye, M. A., & Kanyoro, R. A. (Eds.). (1992). *The will to arise: Women, tradition, and the church in Africa*. Maryknoll/NY: Orbis Books.

Patterson, A. (2011). *The church and AIDS in Africa: The politics of ambiguity*. Boulder, CO: First Forum Press.

Pearson, M. (2010). *DFID Malawi impact evaluation of the SWAp*. DFID.

Philpot, D. (2004). The Catholic wave. *Journal of Democracy, 15*(2), 32–46.

Phiri, I. A. (1998). The initiation of Chewa women of Malawi: A Presbyterian women's perspective'. In J. L. Cox (Ed.), *Rites of passage in contemporary Africa: Interaction between Christian and African traditional religions*. Cardiff: Cardiff Academic Press.

Rankin, S. H., Lindgren, T., Rankin, W. W., & Ng'Oma, J. (2006). Donkey work: Women, religion, and HIV/AIDS in Malawi. *Health Care for Women International, 26*(1), 4–16.

Schatz, E. (2005). 'Take your mat and go!': Rural Malawian women's strategies in the HIV/AIDS era. *Culture, Health and Sexuality, 7*(5), 479–492.

Smith, K. P., & Watkins, S. C. (2005). Perceptions of risk and strategies for prevention: Responses to HIV/AIDS in rural Malawi. *Social Science and Medicine, 60*(3), 649–660.

Soothill, J. E. (2010). The problem with 'women's empowerment': Female religiosity in Ghana's charismatic churches. *Studies in World Christianity, 16*(1), 82–99.

Trinitapoli, J. (2006). Religious responses to aids in sub-Saharan Africa: An examination of religious congregations in rural Malawi. *Review of Religious Research*, 253–270.

Trinitapoli, J. (2009). The Malawi religion project: Data collection and selected analyses. *Demographic Research, 21*(10), 255–288.

Turner, V. W. (1967 [1962]) Betwixt and between: The liminal period in *rites de passage*. In V. W. Turner (Ed.), *The forest of symbols: Aspects of Ndembu ritual* (pp. 93–111). Ithaca: Cornell University Press.

UNAIDS. (2001). *United Nations Declaration on HIV/AIDS at the General Assembly Special Session on HIV/AIDS*.

van Gennep, A. (1960 [1909]). *The rites of passage* (M. B. Vizedom & G. L. Caffee, Trans.). Chicago: University of Chicago Press.

Williams, R. (1976). *Keywords*. London: Picador.

Open Access This chapter is licensed under the terms of the Creative Commons Attribution 4.0 International License (http://creativecommons.org/licenses/by/4.0/), which permits use, sharing, adaptation, distribution and reproduction in any medium or format, as long as you give appropriate credit to the original author(s) and the source, provide a link to the Creative Commons licence and indicate if changes were made.

The images or other third party material in this chapter are included in the chapter's Creative Commons licence, unless indicated otherwise in a credit line to the material. If material is not included in the chapter's Creative Commons licence and your intended use is not permitted by statutory regulation or exceeds the permitted use, you will need to obtain permission directly from the copyright holder.

CHAPTER 6

The Construction of Policy: Donors, AIDS and Cultural Practices

> The 15th International Conference on AIDS took place in Bangkok. Delegates welcomed an increase in funding to combat the disease but disagreed how to spend the money most effectively. Politics rather than science dominated the discussions. (*The Economist*, 17 July 2004)

This chapter explores the dynamics of the policy development process. By focusing on narratives, I show that the policy process is not characterised by rational policymaking but by people's views and interpretations. First, I analyse the process of policy construction. Second, I look at the aid game in Malawi. Third, I look at how these narratives have been passed on through education. Fourth, I present data from interviews I conducted with UNAIDS to present stakeholders' responses to the question *Does your organisation use evidence to inform policy and programmatic decisions on HIV/AIDS?* In my conclusion I reflect on the policymaking process and why policy and programmes on HIV prevention in Malawi are ineffective.

THE PROCESS OF POLICY CONSTRUCTION

In the 1990s we witnessed a great rush to produce global policies on AIDS (see Chapter 4 on international frameworks on AIDS): it was acknowledged that the greatest impact of the AIDS pandemic had taken place in low and middle-income countries, particularly in sub-Saharan Africa. The international AIDS community produced policy documents in abundance, raising and spending millions of pounds on prevention, and although the number of new infections had been falling (UNAIDS 2010) there is not much evidence that policy (Ainsworth and Teokul 2000) nor prevention programmes have been effective (Potts et al. 2008). As Chin argues, HIV prevention programmes have only received limited success (Chin 2007). I present three examples to demonstrate how policy and prevention programmes are not working. Firstly, Ainsworth and Teokul (2000) state:

> [T]here are remarkably few policy success stories on a national scale. Thailand is the clearest case: after an intense national campaign to raise condom use in commercial sex, the condom use rate for brothel-based sex workers reached more than 90%, STD cased declined precipitously, and HIV prevalence among army conscripts dropped by more than half. Infection rates among pregnant women have since declined, although are still high at 1-2%, and these accomplishments seem mostly sustained throughout the East Asian financial crisis. In Uganda, HIV prevalence has declined among pregnant women and young people who are delaying sexual activity. However, it is difficult to attribute either of these outcomes to public policy. The decline in prevalence may be due to heightened mortality among HIV-positive individuals or the natural evolution of human behaviour faced with a generation of high mortality associated with sexual behaviour. (Ainsworth and Teokul 2000, p. 55)

Second, a mathematical modelling tool, known as the modes of transmission model, is used by decision-makers to target measures for preventing HIV infection. The model estimates the number of new HIV infections that will be acquired over the ensuing year by individuals in risk groups that have been identified in a given population using data on the size of the groups, the aggregate risk behaviour in each group, the current prevalence of HIV infection among the sexual or injecting drug partners of individuals in each group and the probability of HIV transmission associated with different risk behaviours (Case et al. 2012). There is evidence from modelling that incidence tended to peak around the mid-late 1990s (Shelton et al. 2006), before much was done regarding HIV prevention. For example, in Malawi the models show incidence peaked in 1997 at 1.91 and by 2011 it was 0.45, but little donor money for AIDS had come into the country before 1997, and the NAC was not formed and active until well after 2000.

Third, money has kept Persons Living With AIDs alive via Anti-Retroviral Therapy, and that might have some prevention impact by lowering viral load, but it is not yet known how much this has contributed to reducing incidence, and in the longer run it might not matter much if inconsistent adherence produces mutations in the virus that cancel these effects.

UNAIDS, a programme established in 1996 by six UN agencies to follow on from the work of the World Health Organisation's Global Programme on AIDS in 1987, was an attempt to coordinate efforts to curb the pandemic. The UN Millennium Declaration, signed by the majority of world leaders, put HIV/AIDS at the top of the international policy agenda. At the first-ever Special Session on HIV/AIDS of the United Nations General Assembly (UNGASS) in 2001, UN Member States strengthened the response to Millennium Development Goal 6 by unanimously endorsing the *Declaration of Commitment on HIV/AIDS*. This *Declaration* included time-bound pledges to generate measurable action and concrete progress in the AIDS response. At the five-year review of the implementation of the *Declaration of Commitment* in 2006, UN Member States reaffirmed the pledges made at the 2001 Special Session. Also, in the *Political Declaration on HIV/AIDS*, they committed to taking action to move towards universal access to HIV prevention, treatment, care and support by 2010 (UNAIDS 2008).

Despite such efforts, the reaction of policymakers in the Global South has been incredibly varied. Some have placed AIDS at the top of the policy agenda and established National AIDS Commissions. However, where National AIDS Commissions have been created the problem has not been fixed (Putzel 2004). Studies refer to the success stories of Senegal and Uganda and claim that infection rates were reduced due to political leadership (Putzel 2003; Moran 2004; Putzel et al. 2006; Foley 2010). South Africa, by contrast, witnessed some of the highest prevalence rates in the world due to the reluctance of politicians to act upon the evidence and respond to the disease. The National Party had 'little incentive to mobilize public resources to counter its impact' (Fourie 2006, p. 52), particularly as the virus appeared primarily in marginalised groups, such as sex workers and white gay men.

The biomedical evidence tells us about the causes of the disease and how to stop it from spreading. It is accepted in global health policy circles that it is sexually transmitted and that it can be prevented by abstinence, mutual fidelity in a partnership that is concordant seronegative or consistent competent condom use. Yet politicians can only take effective action if they take on board the epidemiological characteristics of the virus. The questions that emerge from my research are: (1) Why has the biomedical view failed to dominate the prevention discourses in Malawi? (2) Why has the international policy community strayed from this knowledge and adopted the narratives of blame constructed by the elite in Malawi?

In most countries in the Global South, AIDS is on the policy agenda. In Malawi policies and programmes on AIDS and sexual cultural practices are not informed by evidence. If this is the case in Malawi is it also true elsewhere? Stakeholders and policymakers think they have evidence, as my interviews presented above highlight. For example, data coming from misreporting, from advocacy documents such as those produced by development agencies or from focus groups and surveys that are small scale are then used to quantify large claims about the causes and reasons for Malawi's high transmission rate. There also seems to be an overemphasis on quantitative data and that numbers provide more 'evidence' than qualitative data. A senior manager working for DFID told me: 'DFID pushes numbers. Much more so than we did in the past' (P30). Another respondent working for USAID informed me that a problem was that people do not accept qualitative, ethnographic studies as evidence (P32). However, it is the qualitative analysis of local peoples' perceptions and knowledge around AIDS and attitudes towards sexual behaviour that give us a much more in-depth picture of how prevalent 'at risk' behaviour actually is and offer possible ways of challenging or breaking cycles of transmission.

Local NGOs are asked to generate numbers, which they dutifully do, but the qualitative analysis that seeks to understand why people hold the views they do is rarely done. In other words, the data on transmission are stark, we can accept it is high, but understanding why it is so is left to the Malawian elite to interpret rather than a rigorous process of systematic ethnographic qualitative research. INGOs presented with the data turn to the elites and ask them to explain it; the narratives of blame have thereby been constructed and presented as the 'why' transmission is high. My interviews and analysis show that the international community then accepts these interpretations which in turn take on a certain 'mythical truth' about transmission rates in Malawi. My data reveal that those national actors asked, for example by DFID, to come up with explanations for the high prevalence do so with vested interests—for example and as Chapters 4 and 5 have shown, they are also driven by religious beliefs and/or by financial incentives. It is hardly surprising that the resulting HIV prevention programmes are largely ineffective in curbing transmission—they simply do not get to the root of the problem as defined through and by the biomedical evidence.

The Development Policy Process

What Is Policy?

There are confusingly many different definitions for the word policy. The Oxford English Dictionary (2007) describes policy as 'a course of action adopted or proposed by an organisation or person'. Anderson (1984, p. 3) defines policy as a 'purposive course of action followed by an actor or set of actors'. 'Purposive' suggests that it is goal oriented which encompasses specific solutions to problems as well as frameworks for implementation. Buse et al. (2005, p. 6) describe health policy as embracing 'courses of action (and inaction) that affect the set of institutions, organisations, services and funding arrangements of the health system'. Many scholars stress that policy is inherently political (Foucault 1991), and in some countries, for example France and Spain, the word policy and politics are the same. Policy draws on concepts from several disciplines: economics, history, political science, public administration and sociology and emerged as a sub-discipline in the late 1960s, mainly in the United States.

Development policy has traditionally been seen as a state-led public policy (Hogwood and Gunn 1984; Grindle and Thomas 1991). However, scholars have recognised a shift in the policymaking process, which now involves a larger group of actors (Buse et al. 2005). It is increasingly observed that the policy process landscape is changing and that public policy is not constrained to the government. Different groups—governments, civil society organisations, coalitions, networks, NGOs, the private sector and religious groups as well as national and international media—are important players in policy development. Bilateral, multilateral agencies and NGOs have their own policies and partnerships between the public and private sector take place which also change the policy landscape. It is therefore not surprising that with so many different policies and partnerships that the policy process becomes confusing and muddled and, as a result, programmes are difficult to monitor and evaluate.

The following examples reveal how policy is made among different actors. When I asked a senior manager at DFID in Malawi 'Can you explain how policy is made within DFID at the country level?' she explained:

> It depends on the issue. Sometimes we are leading. Sometimes we are following. DFID buys into the country led approach. It is about what is needed in the country and what the Government of Malawi wants to do on HIV. HIV is a massive problem. So here right now we are continuing with a policy that is already up and running. We continue to monitor a whole set of indicators. We have a key request to disburse £8 million pounds for the Sector Wide Approach. There are gaps regarding challenges and opportunities. Policy is ongoing – you need to check you are on track and you are not missing a trick. (P30)

This passage clearly highlights the extent to which DFID follows and adopts both the policies and explanations behind them already formulated at the national level. She went on to say: 'One thing DFID has done a lot of is trying to solve problems' (P30). DFID sees itself as a trouble shooter swooping into sort out implementation challenges, it does not however seem to take the lead in the design of policy or even the collection of data by which policy may be evidenced.

When I asked the Country Director of World Vision how do they develop policy he said: 'We try to look at government country level policies—like HIV/AIDS. We interpret policies and work "hand in hand". We also work with different donors. We have received money from DFID for work in the past' (P28).

So again, World Vision is admitting here to not taking a lead role in the formulation of policy but rather works with national actors on the implantation of pre-agreed priorities accepting the evidence and narratives put forward by national stakeholders justifying a particular set of actions. Similarly one respondent at USAID told me 'USAID's work depends on the policies of the government' (P31). Once again we see the role of the bilateral and multilateral aid community to be one of supporting and funding implementation not questioning or challenging the wisdom of the national strategies themselves. A policy document entitled 'Malawi –German Health Programme, *Malawi-German cooperation in the health sector*', revealed:

> The Malawian and the German governments cooperate closely in the sectors basic education, democratic decentralisation and health. Malawi-German cooperation with the health sector has a long history going back to the 1980s. Its ultimate goal is to improve the health status of the

population. The German government supports the SWAp as a means of efficiently delivering the range of health services specified under the EHP. (n.d., p. 5)

In my interviews with staff at UNAIDS it was clear that they were unhappy with the operational structures of the Government of Malawi and specifically the way that the national AIDS strategy was put together and presented. Staff told me they felt it had been compiled in a rush with no adherence to participatory methodology that stresses the need for local views and experiences to be gathered systematically feeding into the policymaking process. In fact, on numerous occasions, I heard staff describe the process as 'quick and dirty'. They felt that the involvement of the private sector in the policy process might have resulted in a much more robust and transparent process of programme design. Instead it was unclear how the resulting programmes were put together, and no clear evidence for the narratives around high transmission available. What is interesting and also troubling is why did UNAIDS not question the narratives emerging from the process if they were unhappy with it and if participation was not happening. The UNAIDS Programme Officer said:

> The private sector has no participation in this process. It wasn't like the forum of active participation. Organisations such as MANET+ and NAPHAM had no consistent opinion and there was no advocacy. The forum in which it was done did not influence active participation. It wasn't very well organised. (P59)

This lack of public critical questioning of the policymaking process is apparent according to the INGOs and donors I interviewed and reveals clear apathy on their part. A reluctance to challenge the government, yet clearly privately acknowledged that the policies and frameworks were not robust. Part of this apathy may be due to contradictory views on the role of these agencies, for example according to UNAIDS its remit is as a facilitating agency however when I interviewed a UNAIDS staff member I was told 'UNAIDS prevention strategy has tried to *influence* the national prevention strategy' (UNAIDS consultancy 16 April 2009). This point of view completely contrasts to the view of the Programme Officer, UNAIDS who I also interviewed who said several times that UNAIDS role was to facilitate, not to influence (P25). This confusion provides an explanation as to why national policy processes remain unchallenged and why certain inaccurate narratives then become taken up without the supporting evidence.

Further explanation emerges through the fact that donors are not always in agreement with each other. So there is no united front between the donor community, this in itself is problematic as concerns are not shared. For example, A DFID staff member informed me that:

> There are issues we have with the Global Fund. Donors are disagreeing over basket funding. We have to negotiate with the Ministry of Finance. Different donors have more or less strict rules and then there are the Global Fund's rules. DFID believes in basket funds and SWAps. (P30)

The next section looks at the theoretical models of policymaking.

THE SCHOOLS OF POLICYMAKING

The concept of policy proposes a puzzling mix of frameworks and theories ranging from extremely prescriptive to descriptive (Heclo 1972). Although there are many theories on how policy is made, understanding how the process works has been principally constrained with two opposing approaches to development policy. These can be summarised as follows. On the one hand there is a rational approach to policy, which was pioneered by Laswell in the 1950s (Laswell 1956). This public policy model, also known as the linear or knowledge-driven model or *stages heuristic*, assumes that policy is a one-way process and that policymakers approach issues in a linear fashion while identifying different stages of the process. Significant features of the rational model are a focus on agenda setting, policy formulation, decision-making, implementation and evaluation (Young and Quinn 2002). Foltz describes the rational approach as decision-making that can be carried out in an 'orderly fashion, starting with assessment of the problem, collection of data, synthesis, weighing of the alternatives, selecting objectives and actions and a system to evaluate performance and outcome' (Foltz 1996, p. 210). According to ODI, the rational model assumes a clear separation between fact (based on evidence, science and objective knowledge) and value (seen as a separate issue, dealt with in the political process). The rational model is also seen as prescriptive and presents an 'ideal model' of how policymaking should happen, providing a way of ameliorating the effectiveness of policymaking through the identification of values and goals before making policy choices and opting for the best policy options based on information regarding the costs and consequence of each (Simon 1957). This model was also seen as the solution to fixing political problems faced by public administrators. Gordon et al. propose that the linear model is 'a normative model and a "dignified" myth which often shared by policy-makers themselves' (1993, p. 8, cited by, Shore and Wright 1997). As Mosse points out:

> Now extensive literature argues that development's rational models achieve cognitive control and social regulation; they enhance state capacity and expand bureaucratic control (particularly over marginal areas and people); they reproduce hierarchies of knowledge (scientific over indigenous) and society (developer over 'to be developed') and they fragment, subjugate, silence or erase the local, all the while 'whisk[ing] these political effects out of sight' through technical discourses that naturalize poverty and objectify the poor and depoliticize development. (Mosse 2004, p. 4)

Nonetheless such approaches continue to be perpetuated as part of the policy development and planning techniques of international development agencies which have encouraged non governmental agencies and governments to use them. Yet this type of framework fails to recognise the gap between theory and practice and many scholars have attacked the rational approach. Sabatier (2007) criticises this model as it presumes a linearity to the public policy process that does not exist in reality, it posits neat demarcations between stages that are obfuscated in practice, and suggests no propositions on causality. In a report for ODI, the UK's independent think tank on international development and humanitarian issues, Young and Mendizabal (2009) concludes that 'more evidence-based development policy may not be possible with traditional linear tools and approaches' (p. 3). In other words, the linear nature of such models is blocking the path for evidence-based policy. Linear tools used in development planning include the logical framework which is a management tool mainly used in the design, M&E of international development projects. Authors sum up problems with the Logframe Approach (LFA):

> Unfortunately (for the logical framework approach at least) we are not working with such a self-contained system and there are so many factors involved which lie beyond the scope of the planned initiative that will change the way things work. Although the LFA makes some attempt to capture these through the consideration of the risks and assumptions, these are limited by the imagination and experience of those involved. As a result

the LFA tends to be one-dimensional and fails to reflect the messy realities facing development actors. (Bakewell and Garbutt 2005, p. 12).

Some scholars talk about the 'non-linearity' of policy where policy is often contested, reshaped or initiated from different points between macro and micro levels (Lipsky 1980; Lindblom 1980; Shore and Wright 1997). On the other hand there is an *incrementalist* view which, as a criticism to the rational model of the policy process, the *incrementalist model* was put forward. The principle advocate of this model is Lindblom (1959, cited by Walt and Gilson 1994) who is concerned with the process of bargaining between different interest groups in the course of policymaking. This model also assumes incremental changes are made over time in order to decrease uncertainty, conflict and complexity in processes of policy change and has descriptive overtones. It is incremental in that the process does not commence with objectives but with what exists and how one can proceed from this point.

However, literature on policy processes is now shifting away from the linear and incremental model and demonstrates such frameworks to be an inadequate reflection of policymaking in practice (Clay and Shaffer 1994; Hajer 1995; Keeley and Scoones 1999). There is a third alternative to these models, and the view that I follow, which looks at the policy process consisting of power dynamics, relationships and vested interests of actors who are driven and constrained by the contexts within which they operate. My view gained from my professional experience working as a Consultant to governments and organisations on strategic planning and policy development resonates with recent literature, which emphasises the complex and messy processes by which policies are understood, formulated and implemented and the range of competing actors' interests involved (Keeley and Scoones 2003). Clay and Shaffer's 1984 book, *Room for Manoeuvre,* describe 'the whole life of policy as a chaos of purposes and accidents. It is not at all a matter of the rational implementation of the so-called decisions through selected strategies' (cited by, Keeley and Scoones 1999, p. 33). Walt and Gilson (1994) observe that rarely scholars look at the process of policymaking, the actors involved and the context in which those actors operate, but instead focus on content. Ramalingam et al. (2008) describe the process as nonlinear and complex with a multitude of factors involved. Keeley and Scoones (2000, p. 4) argue that this complexity 'may allow spaces for the assertion of alternative storylines and practices, which, in turn, can gradually result in substantial challenges or shifts in the knowledge and practices associated with previously dominant discourses'. This can be seen in the Malawian context where the process is complex due to the amount of actors involved in policymaking.

Keeley and Scoones (1999, 2003) suggest that policymaking requires three broad *approaches*. One, policy emphasises political economy and interaction of state and civil society and different interest groups. Two, it examines histories and practices linked to shifting discourse and three, it gives primacy to roles and agency of individual actors. There is an integration of different but overlapping perspectives, rooted in different schools of thought and disciplines, which explore how actors make and shape policy narratives and interests while at the same time being constrained. McGee (2004) talks of the 'unpacking' of policy by looking at three different *concepts*: actors, knowledge and spaces. IDS (2006) adopt a similar conceptual framework to analyse the policy process but refer to three interconnected *themes*, namely discourse/narratives; actors/networks and politics/interests. It is important to note that the policy process does not take place in a void. Rather it takes place within a context in which history, culture, political economy, politics and power relations shape aspects of the context, the policy spaces and the way actors and knowledge interrelate to them (McGee 2004, p. 23).

The role of NGOs in the policy process compared to district governments is often confusing as I discovered (Box 6.1). Save the Children was once the umbrella organisation in Balaka and was responsible for distributing funds. Then the Government changed the system and put the district government in charge of funding CBOs. Officials were sent from NAC headquarters in Lilongwe to provide training to CBOs on proposal writing to secure funds. What I then found was that the proposals submitted by the CBOs and FBOS after NAC officers had provided training on proposal writing the majority of CBOs were asking for funds to work on eradicating cultural practices. This has to be questioned as to why most CBOs that had different organisational objectives would be requesting funds for eradicating sexual cultural practices. For example, I obtained the proposals from Balaka District Council and it was clear from my analysis of them that the current trend at the time focused on the eradication of HCPs and CBOs knew that if they asked for money to work on cultural practices and behaviour change they would be more likely to secure it, whether or not they then used these funds on projects focused on eradicating HCPs is not clear, it is possible they diverted funding into their own commitments, through which perhaps a degree of meaningful impact was in fact achieved.

Box 6.1 P15 Interview with a District Youth Officer

S: Okay, let's continue with your work, how do you get funding from the Ministry of Health (MoH), do you get it directly?

R: We get funding from various NGOs, we have the Malawi Bridge project in Lilongwe, we have worked with them they have assisted us in many areas, we are also working with other NGOs like Concern Universal, Self Help Africa, formerly known as Self Help Development International, MACOHA, and there are a lot of NGOs, based in Balaka, they are working in Balaka and Ntcheu. The coordinator is based in Ntcheu; we combine the districts Balaka and Ntcheu. Save the Children, they phased out but we have worked with them, PSI, Blantyre Synod, Sue Lyder foundation, YONECO, Maphunziro foundation.

S: So they give you funding?

R: They don't directly give us funding but they conduct some activities for the youth so we take advantage of them because as government we have the programme and these people know what the government want to do with the youth. They realize that the government itself cannot manage to do all these activities; it is also depending on the NGOs.

S: How do they know what the government wants to do?

R: We have stakeholders meeting with them at least once or twice a year

S: With all the NGOs?

R: With all of them and during such meeting we disseminate what the youth policy is all about and its during this stakeholders meeting it's when the NGOs know what the youth policy is all about, say about the youth. So what they are doing it has to be in line with the youth policy.

S: So how does it work?

R: If they are not doing what is in line with the youth policy, we have to tell them that no, this is not what the youth policy says about the youth, this is what you are supposed to be doing.

S: So do they do their activities independently?

R: Of course they can do things independently but they have to follow what is in the youth policy

S: So does the youth policy mention about cultural practices?

R: Yes, it mentions about the cultural practices, I had a copy but somebody took it last week.

S: And the other NGOs, how do they know about trying to change cultural practices?

> R: Let's go back to the youth... I mentioned about the cultural practices that enhance the spread of HIV/AIDS among the youth, there is a mention of that.
> S: Okay, how do you work with the NGOs and how do you make sure that what the NGOs are doing is in line with the national policy?
> R: When they are implementing their activities, they inform us that this is what we want to do with the youth and we go and see their project and we sometimes advise them on how they can go about it, sometimes they invite us, say, come and see what we are doing, or before they start the programme, they invite us to see what they are doing, but there are some who are implementing youth activities without informing our office, that is an offence, if we discover them, it's an offence.
> S: What do you do?
> R: We sue them and we tell them to come and brief us on what they are doing, if they continue doing that then we sometimes, we have what we call the district executive committee. This is the committee for all heads of government and NGOs, we have that in Zomba. In this committee all the activities that are happening in the district are briefed there so if an NGO is found doing what is not in line with government policy then it's taken to task. But people are careful; they know that if we do what is not in line with what the government wants to be done. So they are much more careful about that.

I spoke to a director of an NGO in Zomba who said his organisation focused on education but he said when speaking to senior managers in charge of NGOs if staff were not personally interested in education then they would not fund projects on this topic. This is an example not just of the institutions objectives but the staff that work for the institutions. If they have personal interests in a specific issue they will not fund projects that want to address other issues even though this issue says education is important and needed in that area. This example demonstrates that even if an organisation has a strategy to implement staff working for the organisation have their own interests and can decide what will be funded. What then is the point of an organisation's strategic objectives if personal interests can get in the way?

CBOs in Malawi are often run by individuals who are motivated by a single set of community rooted issues, they will manipulate their own agenda in order to secure funds but ultimately are unwilling to side-track from their priority. Much money intended for HIV/AIDS was channelled through CBOs who were contracted to use it to eradicate HCPs, the lack of transparency in the process makes it difficult to know if this happened. For example, when I analysed 43 funding proposals submitted by CBOs to Balaka District Council for projects on harmful cultural practices and HIV/AIDS I found that although the project proposal stipulated they would be working on HIV/AIDS when I looked at the budget I discovered that the activities they wanted to fund were related to income generation which suggest these funds were being re-diverted for other projects which the CBO heads felt were of greater priority. These projects not only did not focus on HCP eradication but did not focus on HIV/AIDS either. The reality of this funding chain and the competing interests and priorities of each link is another key factor why donor money failed to have any dramatic impact in reversing transmission rates in Malawi.

The relationship between CBOs and INGOs in Malawi is fraught with tensions. INGOs are essentially donors who wield great power in determining how and which CBOs receives funding. As Lewis and Kanji pointedly describe:

> For post-development critics such as Temple (1997), NGOs are viewed negatively as a continuation of colonial missionary traditions and as the handmaidens of the capitalist destruction of non-Western societies. Within this view, NGOs are modernizers and destroyers of local economies and communities which were once based on age-old systems of reciprocity, into which NGOs introduce undesirable Western values. (2009, p. 44)

Locally based CBOs in Malawi have found a way around the power hierarchy of the aid industry, they play the game to an extent, securing funding and then continue as they please, whether or not their efforts bring about positive development outcomes has not been closely explored as demonstrated above by my analysis of funding proposals submitted to Balaka District Council by CBOs.

CBO employees know how to play the donor game. But the 'big' donors who sit in their offices in the capital rarely meet the CBOs, at least not in the field, therefore have no idea what is actually needed on the ground in the villages. When I interviewed the health specialist at DFID he had been in situ for four months and he could not talk about cultural practices even though DFID had funded a project on cultural practices and were funding national NGOs and the NAC who were distributing funds to CBOs to work on 'sensitsing religious and traditional leaders' about the eradication of cultural practices which were, according to the narrative, spreading the HIV virus. Although he could not talk about the things that were being funded he volunteered to talk about 'policy'. He said:

> NGOs, CBOS and MOH and NAC have had a role in the grant making process which is a national agreement. We support other organisations and international NGOs; for example, the Malawi Economic Justice Network. We have the right focus to ensure vulnerable groups are properly taken into account. (P4)

He then said he can get very absorbed in the process. He also said that DFID ensures that they (DFID) are aware of impact. Although DFID may be aware of impact through reporting procedures I discovered that there seems to be a disconnect between the donors and the CBOs that actually carry out the work, which seems to largely work to the advantage of local organisations who can carry on without fear of scrutiny with the agenda they themselves have set.

INGOs working in line with the government's national strategy put together training and capacity building workshops in order to help CBOs deliver and achieve on the goals of HIV/AIDS eradication (Webb 2004). As an academic pointed out who worked at the College of Medicine:

> Where is the evidence? When policy was developed people did not know how HIV was spread. The perception was that if you had sex with someone who is HIV positive then you would be infected. However 20 years later epidemiologists have discovered that there is 1 in 1,000 chance of contracting HIV. (P50)

This reaffirms my point that evidence is not being used to implement policies and programmes on HIV/AIDS prevention in Malawi. Projects are funded because certain topics become the trend in the development field and the latest topic that donors want to prioritise. Yet if donors choose to increase funding for a particular issue they must decrease funding for other issues unless they can obtain additional resources (Feeny and McGillivray 2004). This can be seen in the case of HIV/AIDS funding. Shiffman (2008) found that donor prioritisation of HIV/AIDS treatment and prevention in developing countries displaced aid for other health issues. UNAIDS reported that:

> It is an unfortunate reality that budgeting procedures too often may mean that new funds for HIV/AIDS can draw resources away from other activities, either at country level, or at donor level. Therefore, all parties need to commit themselves to the principle that additional funding for HIV/AIDS is to be used for additional spending, otherwise displacement is inevitable to the detriment of overall development. (UNAIDS 2004, p. 145)

A study carried out in Malawi which looked at local people's needs revealed that villagers' main concern was not HIV/AIDS but water. Here we see a discrepancy between international policy and the reality on the ground, and how donors are not in tune with what is really needed (Dionne 2011). Ironically, and from my observations and conversations with CBOs in Malawi, it is likely that HIV/AIDS money, at least some of it, is being used to meet these more immediately perceived needs.

What I have demonstrated so far in this chapter is that policy is confusing. Who is implementing what and from what direction? (See my analytical framework.) As I have evidenced in the light of my conversations I have presented in this chapter it is difficult to identify who is making the policy decisions in the development arena because there are so many actors involved in the process. The next section looks at actors' roles as actors are key to the policymaking process.

Actors

Some authors use the term actors to refer to people, others include collectivities such as organisations or government. The term includes politicians, central government officials, local government officers, civil society organisations, NGOs and technical experts. Increasingly, new actors enter the policy process, perhaps by invitation to demonstrate stakeholder participation by those who are holding power, or for their own vested interests. Indeed, actors have vested interests; they are rooted in political and institutional cultures and they make use of agency. As demonstrated in Chapter 3 actors are constantly entering or leaving the development arena and they may have a diversity of vested interests to pursue their own agendas, as well as representing an organisation; a pertinent point which is rarely documented by the international donor community (Kaler and Watkins 2001; Luke and Watkins 2002; Dorman 2005; Marsland 2006).

Actors have the potential to wield enormous power over policies and programmes as they produce their own interpretations of knowledge and thereby construct and influence policy. This can happen at the local, national or international level. The power of actors (agents) is often woven with the structures (organisations) to which they belong. One person told me that if initiation ceremonies were eradicated then key actors involved in the process would lose their jobs such as the initiation counsellor and the hyena. For the actors involved it is an economic activity; the initiation counsellors can earn between 3000 and 5000 kwacha (6–10 pounds) per initiation. Another person said: 'If the cultural practices were removed there would be no research to conduct and then the researchers would lose their jobs' (P44).

Actors are those who have some role in the policy process. As Brock et al. (2001, p. 3) highlight: 'an approach to policy processes that puts actors into the picture has much to offer in making sense of poverty policy processes'.

The policy process involves a complex web of interactions between a range of actors who are strategically positioned in the AIDS arena. The rise and fall of different policy emphases depend upon the ability to underpin narratives to galvanise ideas and people around positions. Policy—built on successful (or otherwise) enrolment of actors—and the creation of networks that are able to make use of policy space emerging from contexts, circumstances and timing. Latour argues that development policy ideas are important less for what they say than for *who* they bring together; what alliances, coalitions and consensuses they allow, both within and between organisations (Latour 1996, pp. 42–43).

What Is Knowledge?

There are different ways of understanding knowledge and therefore different types of knowledge. According to Keeley and Scoones: 'knowledge is produced discursively: it reflects and shapes particular institutional and political practices and ways of describing the world' (Keeley and Scoones 2000, p. 3). When trying to gain knowledge the social sciences tend to oscillate between two opposing concepts: positivism and constructivism. These concepts are linked to assumptions about ontology, epistemology and the philosophy of science. In this positivist versus constructivist war one of the disputes is whether human behaviour is 'caused' by factors external to the individual or whether a person is a participating and, in principle, freely deciding member of a culture and society (Whimster 2007). Whereas positivists can be seen as 'explainers' of reality by emphasising empiricist observation based on rational decisions, constructivists are more concerned with meaning and 'verstehen' (understanding). These 'paired oppositions' as Bourdieu (1988, p. 778) explains, 'construct reality...*they construct the instruments of construction of reality:* theories, conceptual schemes, questionnaires, data sets, statistical techniques, and so on'.

The social construction of policy is made up of narratives and discourses and is irrational. Roe uses the term 'development narratives' and holds the view that narratives are stories or arguments which have a beginning, a middle and an end and revolve around a sequence of events or positions in which something happens or from which something follows' (Roe 2005, p. 314). Keeley and Scoones (2000) uphold that narratives are shaped by the policy process and also shape the way those involved in the policy process act. ODI indicate that narratives define a problem, explain how it comes about and show what needs to be done. Further validity is often gained despite the fact complex issues and processes are frequently simplified.

Discourses, however, according to Hajer, are defined as 'a specific ensemble of ideas, concepts and categorisations which are produced, reproduced and transformed in a particular set of practices and through which meaning is given to physical and social realities' (Hajer 1995, p. 44). For Roe (1991) discourses separate the way problems are thought about, connecting different issues often in highly programmatic, narrative, cause and effect form. These discourses and the institutional practices which they depend on are frequently so embedded that people are unaware of them and they form world views (Keeley and Scoones 2000). As Gasper and Apthorpe (1996) indicate, 'discourse' is understood and used in a range of different ways in the policy process literature.

Foucault (1979), who argues for the strategic reversibility of discourse, suggests:

> There is not, on the one side, a discourse of power and opposite it, another discourse that runs counter to it. Discourses are tactical elements or blocks operating in the field of force relations; there can exist different and even contradictory discourses within the same strategy; they can, on

the contrary, circulate without changing their form from one strategy to another, opposing strategy. (1979, pp. 101–102)

This is an important point as it relates to my research in that discourses on HIV/AIDS and cultural practices are being used to accuse those living in rural areas as being backwards and spreading the disease and that these practices need to be eradicated thereby creating employment opportunities for themselves.

NETWORKS

The AIDS prevention community in Malawi is a network of professionals. Such networks are able to create knowledge and formulate policies. AIDS prevention network I focused on comprised NGOs, INGOs, local and national government, universities and bi and multilateral donors. There have been many different definitions to describe these networks. Castell (1996) describes them as a network society. Haas' (1992) notion of the 'epistemic community' is particularly useful for conceptualising the HIV/AIDS prevention community in Malawi; Haas describes an epistemic community as 'a network of professionals with recognised expertise and competence in a particular domain or issue-area' (Haas 1992, p. 3). He posits that epistemic communities are groups of professionals, often from a variety of different disciplines, which produce policy-relevant knowledge about complex technical issues (Haas 1992, p. 16). Such communities embody a belief system around an issue which contain four knowledge elements: (1) a shared set of normative and principled beliefs, which provide a value-based rationale for the social action of community members; (2) shared causal beliefs which are derived from their analysis of practices leading or contributing to a central set of problems in their domain and which then serve as the basis for elucidating the multiple linkages between possible policy actions and desired outcomes; (3) shared notions of validity—that is, intersubjective, internally defined criteria for weighing and validating knowledge in the domain of their expertise; and (4) a common policy enterprise—that is, a set of common practices associated with a set of problems to which their professional competence is directed, presumably out of the conviction that human welfare will be enhanced as a consequence (Haas 1992, p. 3).

It is important to understand which actors set the debates and influence policy. A senior DFID staff member informed me: 'I have two health advisers. You met with John and are trying to hook up with Sandra. They are part of a network of professionals' (P30) and evaluators of the curriculum books included staff from USAID, UNFPA and the Ministry of Education. Staff from the UN agencies were described as 'expert judges'. These examples illustrate how those working for bi and multilateral donors are given elevated titles such as 'experts' and 'professionals' thus demonstrating their apparent expertise among the donor community. Yet their expert knowledge does not extend to understanding the local contexts which the policy endorsed intends to change. In other words, they have not spent any time gathering local contextual knowledge of AIDS.

Knowledge is constructed in policy and human beings are not blank sheets, hence knowledge is filtered through preconceived ideas and values. Thus it is not an accumulation of facts but involves ways of construing the world. Scientific evidence can be sought to justify a particular policy position however actors are able to cherry-pick points to justify their arguments. As a result policy processes include some perspectives and exclude others, often of the poor and marginalised. Policymakers can also frame scientific enquiry as I have demonstrated in this thesis. Science has been framed in the context of sexual cultural practices spreading HIV/AIDS. A combination of science and policy then plays down scientific uncertainties. Knowledge has been used in international development policy however it is important to ask how has the knowledge been gathered? Often in development, knowledge has been gathered by top-down methods and controlled by national or international elites. Local events are then being reinterpreted or reconstructed within international frameworks. Narratives about HIV policy become normalised. Discourses about harmful cultural practices in Malawi circulate so that people assume the practice is contributing to the spread of HIV but to what extent no one actually knows. One example illustrates my argument. I interviewed a Programme Officer working for UNAIDS and she said:

> We've talked about the cultural practices, we have people talking about it but we don't really have evidence about what is happening in each district, but we've been told and informed by the communities, the leaders within the communities, that yes it is happening. You know, the government people, the NGOs that are working there, they are saying 'yes they are happening'. But we really want to have substantial information for us to be able to say 'yes it's an issue and we need to do something about it. (P25)

This is an example of how evidence is not being used to support policy decisions. Keeley and Scoones (2000) point out that analysis of the policy process requires an examination of how discourses are created and supported through institutions of science, government and administration and to find out where they are contested, where they are open to incremental change and where alternative discourses are emerging and finding expression in the policy process. The concept of 'space' is used in literature on policy change (Brock and McGee 2002) and citizen participation (Jones and Gaventa 2002). Conceptualising policy arenas as 'spaces' where different discourses and actors interact builds on the influential work of Grindle and Thomas (1991). They describe policy spaces as interventions or events which create new opportunities and reconfigure relationships between actors or bring in new ones. This can be seen in the case of Malawi where stakeholders come and go: new ones enter the HIV/AIDS prevention arena where others leave and move on to different jobs in the development field. Hajer talks about 'new spaces of politics' where there are 'concrete challenges to the practices of policy-making and politics coming from below' (Hajer et al. 2003, p. 8). In their view, policy has become more deliberative: less top-down, involving networks and more interpretative, taking on board people's narratives, their understandings, values and beliefs revealed through language and behaviour. This is the view that I also hold which is policy is made on the basis of people's beliefs and not on scientific evidence. Spaces can be categorised in a number of ways. Jones identifies two dimensions: the level and the place and the forms of power maintained within them (Jones et al. 2009). Gaventa (2006) argues that the ways in which spaces are created also play a pivotal role: spaces can be closed, made by a set of actors behind closed doors; invited, where efforts are made to widen participation with citizens groups invited to participate; or, claimed, where less powerful actors create spaces or claim them against the power holder, often emerging out of common concerns or identifications.

Drawing on the conceptual work by Cornwall (2002) and Jones & Gaventa (2002), McGee identifies five dimensions that make up a policy space: history, access, mechanics, dynamics and learning dimensions. She argues that these are pivotal factors for consideration by policy actors considering engagement or analysts trying to comprehend what drives certain episodes or outcomes of policy processes (McGee 2004, p. 18). Another typology categorises spaces according to their functions in the policy process: conceptual spaces (where new ideas are introduced), bureaucratic spaces (formal policymaking led by civil servants), invited spaces (where new ideas are introduced), bureaucratic spaces (formal policymaking led by civil servants), invited spaces (such as consultations), popular spaces (such as protests and social movements), practical spaces (providing opportunities for 'witnessing' by policymakers) and political/electoral spaces (elections) (KNOTS 2006, cited by, Jones et al. 2009). These frameworks on policy spaces have helped my argument as what can be seen in the case of Malawi is certain stakeholders are invited to certain spaces (e.g., meetings) but not others (see UNAIDS example provided earlier regarding participation of the private sector) to develop policy.

One study by Wachira and Ruger (2011) presents findings on the impact of the PRSP process on Malawi's National HIV/AIDS Strategic Framework (NSF). In 2007, a survey was carried out which sought respondents' retrospective perceptions of NSF resource levels, participation, inclusion and governance before, during and after Malawi's PRSP process (2000–2004). Malawian government ministries, United Nations agencies, members of the Country Coordination Mechanism, NAC and NAC grantees were interviewed ($n=125$, 90% response rate). The authors of the article also assessed the principle health sector and economic indicators and budget allocations for HIV/AIDS. Results of the survey suggested that the PRSP process supported accountability for NSF resources but that the process may have marginalised key stakeholders, potentially undercutting the implementation of HIV/AIDS Action Plans. In section "The Development Policy Process" I will now present the case of Malawi using the analytical framework in order to analyse the policy process.

THE AID GAME

Donors' choice of a particular form of aid (relief, bilateral or multilateral development, policy-based or project-based assistance) reflects their global policy objectives and their analysis of how aid contributes to the development process. As development theories change and circumstances in affected countries alter, so donors have increased or decreased the proportion of their aid channelled through the state in recipient countries—the greater the international legitimacy of a recipient country's government, the more bilateral and developmental the channels of assistance are likely to be (Crewe and Young 2002). Donors' choice of aid instrument is also affected by the degree to which they wish to engage with the recipient state (Macrae 2001).

Donors are increasingly moving away from providing financial support to UN agencies in favour of NGOs working through field offices in country. For example, DFID provides funding to more than 100 UK civil society organisations as well as organisations in developing countries. The 'aid chain' (Bebbington 2005) can then be very long which makes it more difficult to monitor and evaluate the impact of the funded programmes. It also makes it harder to uncover how policy and funding decisions were/are made. This can be seen in the case of Malawi. Three examples of the aid chain are: (1) DFID in Malawi funds the NAC, the NAC distributes funds to the district governments and the district governments distribute funds to community-based organisations. (2) DFID UK distributes the money to an NGO in London, the NGO in London distributes the funds to a national HIV/AIDS NGO in Malawi, the National HIV/AIDS NGO distributes it to hundreds of CBOS in the country. These examples support my argument that donors are supporting projects at many different levels of the aid chain. Although DFID, for example, may know what it is funding through the process of reporting I did not see any evidence that a National HIV/AIDS NGO reports to DFID on every single project a CBO is implementing but instead provides a summary of activities the NGO has funded. These CBOs are in the villages and are tiny. For example, I interviewed a Programme Officer working for UNAIDS she gave an example of how UNAIDS gives funds directly to nationally present NGOs to complement the interventions that UNAIDS is implementing. She said:

> We are giving money to four NGOs in 4 districts (Chitipa, Nsanje, Ntcheu and Mangochi) to help build their capacity and implement some of their activities in relation to harmful cultural practices and HIV/AIDS. We did an expression of interest, some NGOs applied; we wanted to see if indeed if in those districts they are indeed implementing activities on HIV/AIDS and cultural practices. So, those ones have been selected but they have not been informed yet; I, myself, don't even know who they are. But we are giving them funds from this year. We have proposed that, with the Flemish, that we need the mapping of the whole country district by district, of what are the cultural practices in those areas. This is the only intervention, because what we are trying to look at with them is that this (mapping) should precede the intervention to address cultural practices. (P25)

This example demonstrates how decisions are being made to influence policy; that four districts were randomly selected to see if cultural practices take place. This example supports my argument concerning how cultural practices are being blamed for the spread of HIV. It also highlights that in this instance the link between HIV/Aids and Harmful Cultural Practices has been accepted, the donor is requesting data on the prevalence and nature of HCP but is clearly not questioning the link. I believe that this multichain reality adds to the distortion and enables particular narratives to emerge unchallenged and unevidenced. The interview above certainly reveals that this narrative has been accepted by donors. The examples that follow also demonstrate that donors have funded work on sexual cultural practices because they believe them to be a significant factor in spreading HIV/AIDS. Several studies, reports and educational materials have been funded by international donors to identify sexual practices and their link to HIV/AIDS rather than how they supported structural gender inequalities and violence. The following section will present these examples.

One study entitled *A Literature Review to support the Situational Analysis for the National Behaviour Change Interventions Strategy on HIV/AIDS and Sexual and Reproductive Health* Coombes (2001) was conducted by the Liverpool Associates in Tropical Health Ltd with funding from the DFID in the UK. The study's findings, which are relevant to this research, came under the topic 'ceremonies and rituals'. It was stated that cultural practices continue to play an integral part in HIV and STI transmission (p. 93). However, the study did not name specific cultural practices neither did it refer to epidemiological data regarding HIV transmission. So once again we see a link between HIV/AIDS and HCP accepted without clear evidence beyond a narrative provided by the Malawian elite. A second study also funded by DFID in entitled *A Review of Cultural Beliefs and Practices Influencing Sexual and Reproductive Health and Health Seeking Behaviour, in Malawi* (Matinga and McConville 2003) makes a similar automatic link between HIV/AIDS and HCPs. The following extract is taken from the introduction:

> The aim of this brief review was to provide a summary of cultural beliefs and practices in Malawi that may serve as risk factors to sexual and reproductive health (SRH). It is simply the *first step* in a process intended to consider deep-rooted cultural issues in the planning and programming of multi-sectoral activities which are focused on mainstreaming HIV/AIDS

and improving SRH. The need for this first step arose because of the lack of accessible data. The DFID supported MoHP Safe Motherhood Programme (SMP) in the southern region is acknowledged for prompting this review by highlighting the links between beliefs, practices and SRH through a needs-based planning process. The audience for this first step is intended to be those involved in developing the Government of Malawi Sexual and Reproductive Health Programme (SRHP), HIV/AIDS organisations, and those in other sectors working towards a cross-sectoral approach. (Matinga and McConville 2003, p. 1)

This is an example of how DFID as a donor has invested money specifically to look at cultural practices because they believe them to be linked to HIV/AIDS. This report also mentions the *fisi* practice of particular interest to me:

'Hyena' (*fisi*) During the ceremony a man (often an older man) undertakes sexual acts with all the girls). His identity is a secret, but he is known as the 'hyena' (i.e. the hyena that comes out at night. SMP research in Mangochi District also notes that the *fisi* may insert a piece of wood into the girl, mimicking the sexual act, a point reiterated by Chirwa (CSR) who believes that much of the sexual activity is symbolic only. (Matinga and McConville (2003, p. 28)

These examples also demonstrate how DFID is funding work on sexual cultural practices despite the fact sexual cultural practices are not mentioned in DFID Malawi's country strategy paper. What again is not elaborated in this document is the way in which these practices generate a gendered ideology that renders girls inferior to men leaving them vulnerable to violence and oppression. The 'symbolic' impact of these practices referred to in this passage clearly indicates the deep-rooted and often subconscious impact these practices have in shaping attitudes and behaviours towards women. DFID however fail to pick up on this choosing instead to focus on an imagined link between harmful cultural practices and HIV/AIDS.

The following is an example of a contract between the Norwegian Ministry of Foreign Affairs and Oxfam. Here we see the adoption of language which is more nuanced. The use of the term harmful cultural practices is not used but instead harmful sociocultural factors that risk causing HIV.

One academic at the College of Medicine told me to go to NAC as 'they have commissioned most studies on sexual cultural practices including funding the work of NGOs' (P51). When interviewing a Research Officer at NAC (p. 46) he described four research reports to support his view and to provide evidence that cultural practices increase vulnerability to AIDS. What is interesting is to see who funds these studies. Those mentioned were a study conducted by the College of Medicine in Blantyre (2005) funded by the NAC. This study was conducted among three ethnic groups of Malawi (the Yao of Balaka, the Chewa of Mchinji and the Sena of Nsanje) and mapped cultural practices and assessed the influence of these on sexual and reproductive health (SRH) outcomes and HIV transmission. The data analysed in this report were collected using qualitative research methods. The evidence presented in this report was a result of 179 interviews conducted in the three sites. These included key informant interviews with traditional leaders, religious leaders, community elders, parents of new initiates, traditional healers, traditional birth attendants, traditional sex counsellors and religious sex counsellors. In-depth interviews were also conducted with married men and women, new traditional and faith-based initiates, recently married men and women, widows, widow inheritors, widowers, *fisiis*, individuals who refused to be cleansed, widows who refused to be inherited, inherited women and participants in ceremonial dances. Study sites were selected villages in Njolomole in Ntcheu, Makanjira in Mangochi and Ndamera in Nsanje. Selection of these sites was purposive and the research process was guided by advice from the District Commissioners and Traditional Authorities. This report did present biomedical evidence and presented the argument that HIV is difficult to contract. It also stated that:

> It follows from the low transmission probabilities of HIV that the most dangerous cultural practices are heterosexual relationships in which sex is frequent, the partner is likely to be infected, and sex is likely to be unprotected. Conversely, the least dangerous are those in which sex is infrequent, the partner likely to be uninfected, and sex is likely to be protected. Other cultural practices such as traditional healing and circumcision are likely to be risky where the same and unsterilized instrument is used.
> (2005, p. 10)

The above paragraph is interesting because it shows how, despite the fact the report presents the epidemiological evidence, it was still deemed necessary to carry out an in-depth study on cultural practices and AIDS.

A report by the Human Rights Commission of Malawi, funded by the Norwegian Agency for Development Cooperation (NORAD) through UNDP and UNICEF, entitled Cultural Practices and their Impact on the Enjoyment of Human Rights, Particularly the Rights of Women and Children in Malawi was also cited. This report made the link between HIV/AIDS and cultural practices by focusing on the human rights narrative and by holding the view that cultural practices are a violation of women's rights. He listed two further studies described as The Priorities in Local AIDS Control Efforts (PLACE) which is a rapid assessment method for identifying areas likely to have sexual partnership formation patterns capable of spreading and maintaining HIV infection. One was entitled 'An Assessment of Risk Practices and Sites where such Practices take place in the urban areas of Lilongwe and Blantyre Districts' (Kadzandira and Zisiyana 2006) and funded by the US Centres for Disease Control and Prevention. This study included a section referred to 'factors that could be facilitating HIV transmissions in the cities of Lilongwe and Blantyre as reported by other patrons'. The factors listed were ignorance/not valuing condom use; poverty/unemployment/more orphans; promiscuity/high sexual partnerships; lack of sensitisation; too much drinking/smoking joints; high cash flow and social life; high population/mobility; peer pressure and other factors.

A second PLACE study also funded by the Centres for Disease Control and Prevention was conducted in July 2006 'to identify sites, events or locations where risky behaviours take place i.e. where people meet new sexual partners and to assess the reach of HIV prevention interventions in these places' (2006, p. vii). This study took place in Nsanje and the passage below highlights that HCP have been placed into the category of risky sexual behaviour, yet again the medical evidence does not support this:

> The prevalence of HIV/AIDS in Nsanje has remained very high (>30% among sentinel surveillance women) and it is for this reason that NAC with funding from the Centres for Disease Control and Prevention (CDC) commissioned the PLACE study in the district so as to generate information that would help in designing prevention interventions. On sexual practices, sexual cleansing to protect widows/widowers, their families and village clans or their property is still being practiced and there are well structured groups who are hired to perform the function at a fee. (2006, p. 1)

This passage also highlights how people focus on Nsanje as a region. This region has been identified as problematic because of the high HIV prevalence rates therefore a link is made between high observation of harmful cultural practices and assumed high transmission rates. This link is not borne out in the national level statistics on prevalence. During this interview I was also told that policy development begins from such studies mentioned above then a research dissemination meeting takes place followed by a planning meeting to take forward the policy recommendations outlined in the research reports. This statement by the NAC staff member demonstrates how perceptions of sexual cultural practices filter upwards and help shape international development policy. These examples demonstrate that these reports act as evidence convincing policy-makers that they are right to pour money into HIV/AIDS programmes which focus on the eradication of HCPs because the donors cite these reports and evidence them.

In an interview conducted in Balaka with a district youth officer I was told that cultural practices are addressed in the gender policy and to implement the gender policy a project was designed called women-girls HIV/AIDS which was funded by the Global Fund (P14). It then transpired that the policy was developed in Lilongwe and that a UN taskforce came to Malawi and decided the project was important as a key way of bringing HIV/AIDS transmission rates down rather than as a way of improving the position of women. Although the district was implementing the project staff are not informed of the size of the budget but they were given a motorcycle and ten bicycles for peer educators 'who are communicating to the community on issues of gender and HIV/AIDS' (P14) by training peer educators and area development committees. This provides an example of the nature of training, for example the training focused around the need for communities to no longer observe those practices thought to increase HIV/AIDS. The reasoning was not based on the negative impact these practices have on the empowerment of girls but on their supposed link to HIV transmission.

In Malawi's national gender-based violence strategy (2002–2006) it states:

> Special thanks are due to GTZ (Deutsche Gesellschaft fur Technische Zusammenarbeit) for funding a consultant and organising a workshop to solicit the views of stakeholders. Awareness and education programmes on GBV to eliminate harmful cultural practices will directly contribute to

reducing risk for girls and women to become infected with HIV/AIDS. Key activities are mainstreaming gender-based violence issues alongside HIV/AIDS in staff training programmes and workplaces. (2002, p. 3)

This shows how the German technical agency is funding work in Malawi to eliminate harmful cultural practices. I interviewed a Programme Officer working for UNAIDS who linked cultural practices and AIDS. She informed me that the Flemish government is providing funding for a study on cultural practices. She said that UNAIDS then gives the funds to the Government of Malawi to implement the AIDS programme and to work on cultural practices. The Programme Officer informed me that cultural practices 'are major things that are issues within the communities'. She said that 'the Flemish will be interested to know what is the status in terms of culture within the country' (P25). This example shows how an international donor is funding research on cultural practices and AIDS.

When I interviewed a staff member at USAID she told me that the final evaluation of a BRIDGE project was being conducted which addressed cultural practices. BRIDGE is an NGO working on BCI In Malawi which USAID funded and provided technical support. Aims of the evaluation were to assess progress in mitigating the impact of HIV/AIDS in Malawi and identify lessons learned and make recommendations for USAID/Malawi to explore in designing future programmes (USAID 2008). The report refers to 'unhealthy cultural practices'. She said that in terms of initiation rites the Traditional Authority still continued with the ceremony but changed it in light of HIV/AIDS. Others also reported how the practice was changed in light of HIV/AIDS for example condoms are used or the act is only symbolic. This highlights the extent to which the primary concern was the risk that harmful cultural practices present to HIV/AIDS rather than the way in which these practices feed into and help maintain patriarchal values. The fact the practices remain even in symbolic form, and that the donor is not concerned to see them eradicated highlights the level of their ignorance in terms of how these practices exacerbate violence towards women. When interviewing the country director, GTZ, I asked if she thought cultural practices contribute to the spread of HIV, she explained:

> Yes of course but you don't see them if you live in Lilongwe or Blantyre. Before I came here as country director I used to come to Malawi and

> visited very, very remote areas to monitor and evaluate programmes. It's a completely different world. Witchcraft takes place and traditional culturally-bound things. (P37)

This comment shows that she thinks cultural practices only take place in remote areas thus reinforcing the views of the Malawian elite I presented in Chapter 4 who try and distance themselves from the high transmission rates by blaming 'the backward culture' of rural communities. However, this is not the case as witchcraft and other forms of African Traditional including traditional healing and medicine also take place in urban areas (Englund 2002). This interview highlights the way that this perception of a backward rural 'other' has influenced and shaped the views of at least some members of the international donor community. She goes on to talk about cultural practices:

> Cultural practices can be disasters for example if you can't get pregnant. Not in Lilongwe or Blantyre but if you cannot get pregnant you would go to a traditional healer. Some of the traditional leaders would contribute to the spread of the disease and would bring in someone to have sex with the woman. (P37)

As pointed out in Chapter 3 where I presented the epidemiology of AIDS this is medically inaccurate. These are examples of how international donors are funding work on cultural practices. Again we see how donors are funding projects to reduce harmful cultural practices because of the primary link to HIV/AIDS not because they represent forms of gender-based violence. So how do these distorted perceptions become so dominant in the international donor community?

Donors Must Get Out More

Donors cover a huge range of organisations; some spend huge amounts of time in the field (e.g., INGOs with country offices), others never visit (e.g., Big Lottery Fund), while others are in between (e.g., DFID staff). However based on my findings a fundamental aspect is the lack of evidence and the fact that donors that are based in the capital of Malawi do not get out into the field often enough means they have a lack of insight into local conditions. Therefore certain donors will accept the views of what goes on in rural communities provided by the Malawian elite whose own agenda was outlined in Chapter 4. For example when I interviewed the HIV/AIDS cluster leader for USAID he said he would like to go out and visit projects more. A DFID officer told me he could not answer any of my questions about sexual cultural practices and had no knowledge about them and said he 'rarely went to the field'. He told me to talk to his Malawian counterpart as he said 'she knows more than me [about cultural practices]'. He also told me he could not talk about cultural practices but could talk about policy. He then went on to say that 'we ensure that we are aware of impact. We think the HIV/AIDS programme is pretty good. Some of it is remarkable' (P4). He also stated that he agreed with the links made between HIV/AIDS and HCP, so despite his willingness to acknowledge he does not go into the field and has no direct understanding—the view on prevalence he puts forward is essentially the narrative of blame constructed by the Malawian elite.

During my consultancy with UNAIDS I asked the question 'How many AIDS-related missions were undertaken by your agency in the last 12 months (either from your headquarters or instigated from the country office)?' The following are some responses (Box 6.2).

Box 6.2   Response to UNAIDS question

"Five in the last six months. So ten. It is our plan to improve this. We are weak on these kinds of missions. We attend conferences and workshops but not real, real missions."

UNAIDS Office, 16/04/09

"Six."

United States Group [USG] Country Coordinator for US Government AIDS Programme PEPFAR 29/04/2009

"We keep a log for incoming missions and they come and support those areas that we itemised. Missions are not instigated by HQ or head office."

Request from Ministry. WHO 29/03/2009

"We have district based staff so we make visits twice every month."

Thomas Kisimbi, Country Director, Clinton Foundation 17/04/2009

"Finances, one per month_____one per quarter."

Director MBCA

"We have contributed a lot and received recognition from NAC to see the work we are doing. We have visited thousands of organisations are visited. Irish Aid also funds some of our work. Not specifically speak about HIV/AIDS but different components Irish Aid mission. Great interest in our work. Help to guide us in terms of what are the best practices out there. Cross cutting issues about gender rights tremendous added value to our work. So I would not be able to quantify the exact number of times".

Concern Universal 20/04/2009

"Yes the National AIDS Commission comes once a year but then they came three times to look at the construction work taking place for the new lecture theatres".

College of Medicine 22/04/2009

"Five in country mission in March from HQ but in the last twelve months we have had two in country missions."

EU office, 16/04/2009

"Two Irish Aid delegates and the Irish Ambassador have visited the programmes in Nsanje district."

GOAL MALAWI

"No visits."

Former HIV and AIDS Coordinator,

GTZ, 12 /05/2009

"So many times. NAC, DFID, Scottish Executive and BRIDGE".

MANASO 20/04/2009

"2 times" Mwanza district 30/04/2009

"6 times" Toveraine 30/04/2009

How Narratives Have Been Passed on Through Education

The narratives of blame also feed into the education system via the curriculum. Curriculum-based education books are used by teachers in schools in Malawi to teach students about developing life skills. UNFPA, NORAD and Swedish International Development Agency (SIDA) funded the development of these text books. I analysed a complete set (2002, 2004, 2008). In 2002 cultural practices were referred to and described as both helpful and harmful. This book referred less to HIV/AIDS. In 2004–2008 however more references were made to harmful practices and HIV/AIDS. Pertinent issues featured in these books were cultural practices and HIV/AIDS, gender and HIV/AIDS and human rights and HIV/AIDS.

In the senior secondary life skills education student's book (Fabiano 2002) cultural practices are reported to encourage the spread of HIV/AIDS. An activity section on 'harmful cultural practices' asks students to:

- Brainstorm cultural practices,
- Work in groups to identify cultural practices which are harmful and those which are not harmful,
- Report your findings to class for discussion,
- Discuss in groups practical solutions to each of the harmful cultural practices, and
- Report your findings to class for discussion.

Cultural practices referred to as harmful include *fisi* (hyena), male circumcision, female circumcision, tattooing for beautification or administration of charms, widow inheritance (*chokolo*) and death cleansing (*kuchotsa kufa*). The *fisi* is described as a man from the village who is given the role of sleeping with young girls as part of their initiation into womanhood (Mthanga et al. 2002). What is unclear is why these practices were identified as harmful as there is no explanation as to why they are deemed harmful. Through the curriculum this narrative of blame is being introduced to children shaping the way they see this issue. The textbooks are funded by international donors who see this approach as an important way of challenging HIV/AIDS as it directly focuses on changing behaviour and attitudes (Box 6.3).

> **Box 6.3 Questions for students on cultural practice and HIV/AIDS**
>
> Review questions
> 1. Give three examples of cultural practices that facilitate the spread of HIV/AIDS.
> 2. Give three examples of cultural practices that help in the prevention of HIV transmission
> 3. Explain how each of the examples you have given in (1) facilitates the spread of HIV/AIDS.
> 4. Write an essay on the impact of HIV/AIDS in your community
> 5. Suggest ways of alleviating the impact of HIV/AIDS on the community.
>
> P109
> Review questions
> 1(a) Give three examples of negative effects of foreign culture and technology on indigenous cultural and traditional practices
> (b) Explain the importance of critical thinking before adopting foreign culture and technology.
> 2. Explain the importance of critical thinking before adopting foreign culture and technology.
> 3. Write an essay on the impact of HIV/AIDS on the nation and the world.
> 4. Suggest ways of alleviating the impact of HIV/AIDS on the nation and the world.

The exercises in curriculum-based books mentioned above demonstrate how misconceptions concerning sexual cultural practices and HIV/AIDS are embedded in people's views at an early age. Research shows that well-designed and well-implemented HIV prevention programmes can significantly reduce sexual risk behaviours among young people and schools should be key to supporting effective HIV prevention among youth. However teaching young people about harmful cultural practices will not lead to a reduction in risky sexual behaviour. As I have outlined the damaging impact of HCP is far more nuanced than immediately rendering girls vulnerable to HIV transmission.

In an interview with a civil servant at the Health Education Unit, Lilongwe (P45) I met him at his office in October 2008. He told me that the Salvation Army did work to develop materials on cultural practices and AIDS. He said the *fisi* practice and *kusasa fumbi* exist. He said in the course of learning adult language, adult techniques they get a woman for a boy and a man for girls. He said they are scared that if they don't do it they will experience drying of skin—coarse skin. He said children practice sex but if they have sex with someone who is infected they get infected. He said that the Health Education Unit is producing a manual and is waiting for funds from headquarters to translate into Chichewa and Chitumbuka. The manual describes how to get into communities and address cultural practices and how to approach traditional leaders and convince them to change the practices. The manual includes sections on: types of relationships; relationship with HIV; Approach; What is it? Cultural practices; What can they do? And what are the dangers? He said the manual will be used by 'change agents' in other words, anyone involved in the issues. He said evidence is difficult to come by and what is needed is a control—a community that hasn't made changes and a community that has. He said evidence for this manual was obtained from interviewing Initiated girls and initiated boys in Mulanje. The Health Education Unit used the information from this research to develop materials.

A PowerPoint presentation I was given by the Seventh-day Adventist Church concerning a Clinic & Community Service Initiative of Adventist health services which spoke about an integrated clinic and community HIV/AIDS/STI prevention project was funded by USAID through the Umoyo network. The programme's objectives included creating awareness on the dangers of harmful cultural practices and advocating for the modification of harmful cultural practices. The presentation also listed positive and negative cultural practices as follows (Box 6.4).

Box 6.4   PowerPoint presentation by the Seventh-day Adventist Church

- Positive
1. Lobola
2. Kumeta
3. Chinamwali
4. Chikamwini/ Chitengwa
5. Wife inheritance to a certain extent

- Negative
1. Fisi
2. Polygamy
3. Magolowazi
4. Property grabbing
5. Post menopausal cessation of intercourse
6. Use of herbs to dry out and tighten of vagina

The presentation then outlines the roles played by the Adventist health services and the community (Box 6.5).

Box 6.5   PowerPoint presentation by the Seventh-day Adventist Church Cont

- Adventist Health Services
1. Facilitate focus group discussion on cultural practices that promote the spread of HIV virus.
2. Train Community based HIV counsellors.
3. Introduce VCT services in two of the nine Supervision areas.

- Community
1. Review cultural practices in relation with HIV/AIDS.
2. Modify cultural practices that promotes the spread of HIV virus.

Where Is the Evidence?

This section presents data from the consultancy I conducted with UNAIDS. The question asked to stakeholders involved in HIV/AIDS was *Does your organisation use evidence to inform policy and programmatic decisions on HIV/AIDS?* (Box 6.6).

This section demonstrates that evidence to inform policies and programmes on HIV/AIDS is weak.

Box 6.6   Data from UNAIDS consultancy

Yes   Please provide examples

No   Do you have plans to improve on this in the future? Please give examples

Director of Planning, Ministry of Health 20/04/2009
This is one area that is still a challenge. We are supposed to do this. Monitoring and Evaluation (M&E) is one area where we need to do a little bit more work. In the districts at the health level, for example in rural health centres we have M&E officers. We don't have specialised information so we are grappling with non- trained statisticians.

They know the policy requires a certain quality of information and timeliness of providing that information and also ownership of that information. Like HIV/AIDS, TC has vertical silos that have their people. The programme wants to correct Malawi Integrated Health Survey (MIHS) one guy needs to sit down and address it is an issue for example MIHS timeliness and quality of reporting for evidence based planning. We are using programme information to request the government department to create positions for m and e graduates. This has not yet happened but the request has been made.

Director, MBCA 22/04/1999
Yes it is based on evidence – what is working well with some of our partners. During m and e visits and biannual review meetings. New members study visits looking at best practices.

Alliance One 20/04/2009
Increase in number of employees with STI's necessitated the company to scale up condom use awareness for those that cannot abstain or stick to one partner. Our clinic registered for ART programme having looked at statistics of employees whose health status was deteriorating as a result of being HIV positive. Referring employees for ART to other health facilities e.g The Light House was proving problematic due to the large number of people looking for the same service.

Concern Universal implementing partner 20/04/2009
We do work internally for advocacy at the national level but we have not played an advocacy role to influence policy at the national level. We are trying to influence the extended NAF in terms of what should be some of the priorities we should be focusing on. Within the room 3 organisations from a perspective. Such things are areas that we have tried to influence.

Doctor, College of Medicine 22/04/2009
I suppose we have to say. What constitutes evidence? There is awareness in university of Malawi. HIV is having an impact both in and outside, members of staff. I cannot remember exactly what the source was how many members of staff died as a result of HIV/AIDS. We need to have an HIV/AIDS policy. Distant memory no formal report

or assessment done to inform policy most policies are made with elements of general knowledge. What other institutions may have. Research in my view the gold standard of evidence is the randomised control trial. Observational studies, audits. Type of evidence I have articulated we see what is happening in other parts of the world. Great knowledge.

ESCOM 20/04/09 This one yah what happens is through these M&Es through these surveys. Our HIV/AIDS policy developed in 2001; reviewed in 2006. Provisions of nutritional supplements Living with HIV/AIDS. Incorporate into programme. Employees. As of now providing ARVs into clinic. After revision. Use evidence. After collecting data go through the responses from questionnaires – steering committee – we haven't reached out through the north. Let's do this, coming up with the results. Do presentation with executive mgt outcome of the survey communicate to my employees. Newsletter produced to all employees. Human resources. Member of staff can access.

Questions about HIV/AIDS. The rest don't know.
GOAL HIV/AIDS M&E Manager 27/04/2009
GOAL Malawi conducts KAPB surveys to determine what issues are there on the ground that need to be addressed. For example, in the past year, GOAL Malawi discovered that stigma and discrimination still exists in the communities and then developed specific interventions to reduce stigma and discrimination and also carry out advocacy campaigns.

MANASO 24/04/2009
Yes a number of activities are actually informed by what is coming from our constituencies. Information from them helps us come up with new programmes. Technical support that we provide to the members workshop set up only thirty members. When we saw that people were under-utilising that. We had to ask them why they weren't implementing what they had learnt. 1. Had not understood. 1. Language barrier. Changed our strategy on site technical support all group members would be present. Ten to fifteen members remind each other. Needs driven. Workshops when the needs are similar. Do have national workshops.

MANET+ PROG OFFICER 24/04/2009
Yes. We have done that. Research on stigma and discrimination that has informed the policy. Part of the policy development process. Also one of the challenges we are facing. Donors not much willing to support, research and m and e just looking at implementation. Stigma response. No nationwide study. Evidence base. For us you will see the irony not only reporting to NAC. In terms of the donors that require support. Results. To follow up on how we can deal with the challenges that we face. Not equated with resources. Development partners not ready to support us on results.

Of course HIVOS supporting in terms of m and e. not expect results on the ground. Want the evidence. Want to hear voices. Results on the ground hear a story. Home based care. Dutch humanist comic relief interested in results. Can share USAID. Not just interested in outputs, success stories. What change have you brought. Voices must be reflected. This is what is not in comparison. There is a lot of money come through NAC programmes. Most of work is advocacy. Difficult to measure. Many partners influencing us. Difficult. Combined interventions. Difficult for one organisation to take success. Good to look at the result. That requires resource. Proportion of monitoring. For NAC come up with a three year proposal. Make much sense. Previous implementation. That is the situation on the ground. Come up with another three year strategy. More or less ready just to get what we are presenting. To some extent not ready to face what we are doing. Why is that we are not making significance strides in behaviour change. That awareness not translated into behaviour change. Over what period. Really moved down. Looked at same methodology. Maybe have shifted the goalposts.

Ministry of Education, 28/04/2009
Yes the evidence analysing the capacity of teachers living +. Issues to be discussed there. Report is here. Take to management to react towards problems identified.

Ministry of Local Government, "no" 29/04/2009

> Mzimba district council 29/04/2009
> Yes district HIV/AIDS has affected us all. Something that when we are implementing has to be mainstreamed. For example if we look at BCI in the district most of them like going to South Africa leaving spouses behind. Wife stays does other things. Created situation need to sensitise the communities to let them know it is more serious. Presenting them to the behaviours. Base all activities if we find if that is a problem. HTC week. If people go for htc if they found positive this area going towards levels we need to act urgently.
>
> Mzudza 20/04/2009
> Yes we do that. Chairman at the ministry level.
>
> Toveraine 29/04/2009
> For our programme we go to the field and assess. Quality Assessment sponsored by Umoyo network. Activities based on what we did during that survey.
>
> Any evidence to inform policy decisions? Trocaire conducted an HIV/AIDS scoping study and a gender study. HIV highly subscribed. Trocaire does not have skills or capacity to fill important gap (P27 09/03/2010).

Conclusion

This chapter examines the complexities of the donor funding process, how inaccuracies come into play, and how reality has become distorted; I have evidenced that distortion and looked at how different narratives merge which then hinder the effectiveness of prevention programmes. Policies and programmes are affected as they are not supported by epidemiological evidence. This is why it has been important to talk about the policy process. If the policy process had been dealt with in a different way and evidence was used to support the policy decision then perhaps HIV prevention programmes would be more effective.

REFERENCES

Ainsworth, M., & Teokul, W. (2000). Breaking the silence: Setting realistic priorities for AIDS control in less-developed countries. *The Lancet, 356*(9223), 55–60.
Anderson, J. E. (1984). *Public policymaking: An introduction* (3rd ed.). Boston, MA: Houghton Mifflin.
Bakewell, O., & Garbutt, A. (2005). *The use and abuse of the logical framework approach.* Stockholm: Swedish International Development Cooperation Agency (Sida).
Bebbington, A. (2005). Donor-NGO relations and representations of livelihood in non-governmental aid chains. *World Development, 33*(6), 937–950.
Bourdieu, P. (1988). Vive la crise! For heterodoxy in social science. *Theory and Society, 17*(5), 773–787.
Brock, K., & McGee, R. (Eds.). (2002). *Knowing poverty: Critical reflections on participatory research and policy.* London: Earthscan.
Brock, K., Cornwall, A., & Gaventa, J. (2001). *Power, knowledge and political spaces in the framing of poverty policy.* Sussex, UK: Institute of Development Studies.
Buse, K., Mays, N., & Walt, G. (2005). *Making health policy.* London: Open University Press.
Case, K. K., Ghys, P. D., Gouws, E., Eaton, J. W., Borquez, A., Stover, J., et al. (2012). Understanding the modes of transmission model of new HIV infection and its use in prevention planning. *Bulletin of the World Health Organisation, 90*(11), 831–838A.
Castells, M. (1996). *The rise of the network society.* Oxford, UK: Blackwell.
Chin, J. (2007). *The AIDS pandemic: The collision of epidemiology with political correctness.* Oxford: Radcliffe Publishing.
Clay, E., & Shaffer, B. (Eds.). (1994). *Room for manoeuvre: An exploration of public policy in agriculture and rural development.* London: Heinemann.
College of Medicine. (2005). *Cultural practices related to sexual and reproductive health outcomes and HIV transmission.* Blantyre: College of Medicine.
Coombes, Y. (2001). *A literature review to support the situational analysis for the national behaviour change interventions strategy on HIV/AIDS and sexual and reproductive health.* London: DFID.
Cornwall, A. (2002). *Making spaces, changing places: Situating participation in development.* Sussex, UK: Institute of Development Studies.
Crewe, E., & Young, M. J. (2002). *Bridging research and policy: Context, evidence and links.* London: Overseas Development Institute.
Dionne, K. Y. (2011). Local demand for a global intervention: Policy priorities in the time of AIDS. *World Development, 40*(12), 2468–2477.
Dorman, S. (2005). Studying democratization in Africa: A case study of human rights NGOs in Zimbabwe. In T. Kelsall & J. Igoe (Eds.), *Between a rock and a hard place: African NGOs, donors and the state* (pp. 33–59). Durham, NC: Carolina Academic Press.

Englund, H. (2002). The dead hand of human rights: Contrasting Christianities in post-transition Malawi. *The Journal of Modern African Studies, 38*(4), 579–603.

Fabiano, E. (2002). *Senior secondary science and technology: Students book 3.* Blantyre, Malawi: Macmillan Malawi.

Feeny, S., & McGillivray, M. (2004). Modelling inter-temporal aid allocation: A new application with an emphasis on Papua New Guinea. *Oxford Development Studies, 32*(1), 101–118.

Foley, E. E., & Nguer, R. (2010). Courting success in HIV/AIDS prevention: The challenges of addressing a concentrated epidemic in Senegal. *African Journal of AIDS Research, 9*(4), 325.

Foltz, A. M. (1996). *The policy process.* Geneva: World Health Organization (WHO).

Foucault, M. (1979). *The history of sexuality, vol. I: An introduction.* New York: Random House.

Foucault, M. (1991). *Discipline and punish: The birth of the prison.* London: Penguin.

Fourie, P. (2006). *The political management of HIV/AIDS in South Africa: One burden too many?.* Basingstoke, UK: Palgrave Macmillan.

Gasper, D., & Apthorpe, R. (1996). Discourse analysis and policy discourse. *The European Journal of Development Research, 8,* 1–15.

Gaventa, J. (2006). Finding the spaces for change: A power analysis. *IDS Bulletin, 37*(6), 23–33.

Grindle, M., & Thomas, J. (1991). *Public choices and policy change: The political economy of reform in developing countries.* Baltimore: John Hopkins University Press.

Haas, P. M. (1992). Epistemic communities and international policy coordination: Introduction. *International Organisation, 46*(1), 1–35.

Hajer, M. A. (1995). *The politics of environmental discourse.* Oxford: Oxford University Press.

Hajer, M., Hajer, M. A., & Wagenaar, H. (Eds.). (2003). *Deliberative policy analysis: Understanding governance in the network society.* Cambridge University Press.

Heclo, H. (1972). Policy analysis. *British Journal of Political Science, 2*(1), 83–108.

Hogwood, B. W., & Gunn, L. A. (1984). *Policy analysis for the real world.* Oxford: Oxford University Press.

Institute of Development Studies. (2006). *Understanding policy processes: A review of IDS research on the environment.* Sussex, UK: IDS.

Jones, E., & Gaventa, J. (2002). *Concepts of citizenship: A review.* Sussex, UK: IDS.

Jones, N., Datta, A., & Jones, H. (2009). *Knowledge, policy and power: Six dimensions of the knowledge-development policy interface.* London: Overseas Development Institute (ODI).

Kadzandira, J. M., & Zisiyana, C. (2006). *Assessment of risk practices and sites where such practices take place in the urban areas of Lilongwe and Blantyre districts*. Zomba: Centre for Social Research.

Kaler, A., & Watkins, S. (2001). Disobedient distributors: Street-level bureaucrats and would-be patrons in community based family planning programs in rural Kenya. *Studies in Family Planning, 32*(3), 254–269.

Keeley, J., & Scoones, I. (1999). *Understanding environmental policy processes: A review* (Vol. 89) (IDS Working Paper).

Keeley, J., & Scoones, I. (2000). *Environmental policymaking in Zimbabwe: Discourses, science and politics*. Sussex, UK: IDS.

Keeley, J., & Scoones, I. (2003). *Understanding environmental policy processes: Cases from Africa*. London: Earthscan.

Lasswell, H. D. (1956). *The decision process*. College Park, MD: University of Maryland Press.

Latour, B. (1996). *Aramis, or the love of technology* (C. Porter, Trans.). Cambridge, MA and London: Harvard University Press.

Lewis, D., & Kanji, N. (2009). *Non Governmental Organizations and Development*. Oxon: Routledge.

Lindblom, C. E. (1980). *The policy-making process*. Englewood Cliffs, NJ: Prentice Hall.

Lipsky, M. (1980). *Street-level bureaucracy: Dilemmas of the individual in public service*. New York: Russell Sage.

Luke, N., & Watkins, S. C. (2002). Reactions of developing-country elites to international population policy. *Population and Development Review, 28*(4), 707–733.

Macrae, J. (2001). *Aiding recovery: The crisis of aid in chronic political emergencies*. London: Zed Books.

Marsland, R. (2006). Community participation the Tanzanian way: Conceptual contiguity or power struggle? *Oxford Development Studies, 34*(1), 65–79.

Matinga, P., & McConville, F. (2003). *A review of cultural beliefs and practices influencing sexual and reproductive health and health-seeking behaviour, in Malawi*. Lilongwe: Department for International Development Malawi (DFID).

McGee, R. (2004). Unpacking policy: Actors, knowledge and spaces. In K. Brock, R. McGee, & J. Gaventa (Eds.), *Unpacking policy: Actors, knowledge and spaces in poverty reduction* (pp. 1–26). Kampala: Fountain Press.

Moran, D. (2004). HIV/AIDS, governance and development: The public administration factor. *Public Administration and Development: The International Journal of Management Research and Practice, 24*(1), 7–18.

Mosse, D. (2004). Is good policy unimplementable? Reflections on the ethnography of aid policy and practice. *Development and Change, 35*(4), 639–671.

Mthanga, A. S., Maluwa-Banda, D., Chiziwa, S. E., & Mphande, D. K. (2002). *Senior secondary life skills education, student's book 3 and 4*. Blantyre: Macmillan.

Potts, M., Halperin, D. T., Kirby, D., Swidler, A., Marseille, E., Klausner, J. D., et al. (2008). Reassessing HIV prevention. *Science, 320*(5877), 749–750.

Putzel, J. (2003). *Institutionalising an emergency response: HIV/AIDS and governance in Uganda and Segal.* London: London School of Economics and Political Science (LSE), Crisisstate Research Centre (CSRC).

Putzel, J. (2004). The global fight against AIDS: How adequate are the National Commissions. *Journal of International Development, 16*(8), 1129–1140.

Putzel, J., Denis, P., & Becker, C. (2006). A history of state action: The politics of AIDS in Uganda and Senegal. *The HIV/AIDS epidemic in sub-Saharan Africa in a historical perspective*, pp. 171–184.

Ramalingam, B., Jones, H., Reba, T., & Young, J. (2008). *Exploring the science of complexity: Ideas and implications for development and humanitarian efforts.* London: ODI.

Roe, E. (2005). Development narratives, or making the best of blueprint development. In M. Edelman & A. Haugerud (Eds.), *The anthropology of development and globalization: From classical political economy to contemporary neoliberalism* (pp. 313–322). Oxford, UK and Malden, MA: Blackwell.

Roe, E. (1991). Development narratives, or making the best of blueprint development. *World Development, 19*(4), 287–300.

Sabatier, P. A. (2007). The need for better theories. In P. Sabatier (Ed.), *Theories of the policy process.* Boulder, CO: Westview Press.

Shiffman, J. (2008). Has donor prioritization of HIV/AIDS displaced aid for other health issues? *Health Policy and Planning, 23*(2), 95–100.

Shore, S., & Wright, S. (Eds.). (1997). *Anthropology of policy: Critical perspectives on governance and power.* London and New York: Routledge.

Shelton, J. D., Halperin, D. T., & Wilson, D. (2006). Has global HIV incidence peaked? *The Lancet, 367*(9517), 1120–1122.

Simon, H. A. (1957). A behavioral model of rational choice. In H. A. Simon (Ed.), *Models of man, social and rational: Mathematical essays on rational human behavior in a social setting.* New York: Wiley.

UNAIDS. (2004). *Report on the global AIDS epidemic: Executive summary.* Geneva, Switzerland: UNAIDS.

UNAIDS. (2008). *2008 report on the global AIDS epidemic.* Geneva, Switzerland: UNAIDS.

UNAIDS. (2010). *UNAIDS report on the global AIDS epidemic.* Geneva, Switzerland: UNAIDS.

Wachira, C., & Ruger, J. P. (2011). National poverty reduction strategies and HIV/AIDS governance in Malawi: A preliminary study of shared health governance. *Social Science and Medicine, 72*(12), 1956–1964.

Walt, G., & Gilson, L. (1994). Reforming the health sector in developing countries: The central role of policy analysis. *Health Policy and Planning, 9*(4), 353–370.

Webb, D. (2004). Legitimate actors? The future role for NGOS against HIV/AIDS in sub-Saharan Africa. In N. K. Poku & A. Whiteside (Eds.), *The political economy of AIDs in Africa* (pp.19–32). Hampshire, UK: Ashgate Publishing.

Whimster, S. (2007). *Understanding Weber*. New York: Routledge.

Young, E., & Quinn, L. (2002). *Writing effective public policy papers: A guide to policy advisors in Central and Eastern Europe*. Budapest: LGI.

Young, J., & Mendizabal, E. (2009). Helping researchers become policy entrepreneurs: How to develop engagement strategies for evidence-based policy-making. *Briefing Paper, 53*.

Open Access This chapter is licensed under the terms of the Creative Commons Attribution 4.0 International License (http://creativecommons.org/licenses/by/4.0/), which permits use, sharing, adaptation, distribution and reproduction in any medium or format, as long as you give appropriate credit to the original author(s) and the source, provide a link to the Creative Commons licence and indicate if changes were made.

The images or other third party material in this chapter are included in the chapter's Creative Commons licence, unless indicated otherwise in a credit line to the material. If material is not included in the chapter's Creative Commons licence and your intended use is not permitted by statutory regulation or exceeds the permitted use, you will need to obtain permission directly from the copyright holder.

CHAPTER 7

Conclusion and Recommendations

The focus of this research was to examine how policies and programmes on HIV prevention and the sexual cultural practice of *fisi* have come to be linked. My findings show that policies have been constructed based on inaccurate imaginings of both the sexual behaviour of rural people, who have been primarily blamed for the spread of HIV, and the Malawian elites' and international donors' misunderstanding of the bio-medical evidence surrounding HIV transmission during one heterosexual act. I have shown this by using the example of the *fisi* practice; a practice that involves a man having sex with girls during initiation. Although there are many sexual cultural practices taking place in Malawi, I focused on this practice, as while I was in Malawi working as Programme Manager for a sexual and reproductive health NGO, it was this practice that was recounted to me at length by those working for NGOs and stimulated a desire to learn more.

According to work on sexual cultural practices, they act as a mechanism rendering women inferior to men, and it is this inferiority that renders them vulnerable to violence (Mkamanga 2000; Kamlongera 2007). For example, Anderson (2012) in her study on women's bodies in Malawi, argues that most women who participate in sexual cultural practices are unable to refuse, as within wider society there is an understanding of a universal 'masculine sex-right' where men have the right to make decisions over what can be done with a female body, which makes women vulnerable to violence. Kistner and Nkosi (2003) argue that masculinity has emerged as one of the key factors at the interface between gender-based violence and HIV/AIDS. Thus, we can see that the practice of such sexual acts can lead to women's susceptibility to violence.

This research draws attention to the fact that the probability of infection from one heterosexual act, such as the *fisi* practice, is very low: as reflected in the epidemiological evidence provided in this research (Gray et al. 2001; Powers et al. 2008). In light of this, the thrust of the study is the exposure of misconceptions among development practitioners and policymakers in Malawi concerning AIDS: this misconception is grounded in the view that certain cultural practices are fueling the HIV pandemic in Malawi. This research has predominately focused on revealing how very little if any bio-medical evidence is being used to inform current policies and programmes on AIDS in Malawi. Instead a handful of Harmful Cultural Practices have been targeted as the problem, which has led to a focus on eradicating those deemed dangerous. Yet I found that there is no evidence that the sexual practice of *fisi* has a higher transmission rate than other sexual practices that are common within Malawi. While a *fisi* may be more likely to be HIV positive than the average male, it is the case that intercourse with a *fisi* is usually a single act of intercourse and is far from an everyday occurrence: since intercourse within marriage is much more frequent and the use of condoms in marriage is infrequent (Chimbiri 2007), regular marital relations are thus more likely to lead to infection than intercourse with a *fisi*. For HIV prevention purposes, it would be far more useful to focus on more frequent practices, such as transmission within marriages or stable couples.

In the health sector, the concept of evidence-based policy has gained ground. Yet as I have demonstrated, a lack of capacity to make use of existing data in policy development and programmes imply that inefficiencies in the development process have not been properly identified and addressed. Most HIV prevention programmes in Africa have also arguably had limited impact because the research behind them focused primarily on risk groups, behavioural change models, and flawed understandings of cultural practices and economic conditions (Packard and Epstein 1991; Waterston 1997). In other words, the explanations given by the National AIDS Commission and non-governmental organisations for high rates did not rely enough on biomedical facts but rather on constructed categories of 'at risk' groups which once interrogated, can be seen to be inaccurate.

In this conclusion I bring together the various threads of my argument. First, I summarise the findings and discussion of this research in relation to the themes identified and the analytical frame employed in this study. Second, I present my three key arguments. Third, I contextualise my study in terms of where we are today with AIDS at the global level and within Malawi. Fourth, I demonstrate how this study contributes to academic debates. Finally, I present recommendations.

SUMMARY OF KEY FINDINGS

In Chapter 1, I provide an introduction to the topic including motivation for this research and my methodological approach.

In Chapter 2 I reviewed the literature within the field of anthropology of development, with particular emphasis on the work of Mosse (2011) and Crewe and Harrison (1998). Both demonstrate that many actors are involved in the policy process, which is not linear or straight forward: this makes it hard to unravel by whom these policies are constructed. These scholars demonstrate the usefulness of ethnography as a way of understanding the threads that interlock in the formation of policies and thereby have helped me identify how misconceptions seeped into the policy process in relation to HIV prevention in Malawi; although I do not analyse the policy process elsewhere in sub-Saharan Africa, it is likely to be similar to that of Malawi. They critically analyse the complex relationships of power between global multilateral organisations, donors, governments of resource-poor countries and local communities, and their impact on development projects. They also demonstrate how to critically engage with development practice by combining academic development work with academic writing and reflection therefore they have insights due to their positioning. Their approaches have been instrumental in developing my own analytical framework, as my research looks at how different elites working within the field of AIDS are able to construct policies based on vested agendas and interests.

In Chapter 2 the work of Chin (2007) is also particularly relevant to the central argument of my research, that elites working on HIV and AIDS perpetuate the myth that the *fisi* practice contributes significantly to the spread of HIV in Malawi. I argue that Malawian elites perpetuate this myth to maintain their professional status and to secure external funding from donors for projects on HIV prevention. Chin (2007) argues that UNAIDS and AIDS activists accept certain myths about HIV epidemiology to keep the disease on the political agenda and, by implication, ensure funding and jobs.

In Chapter 2, due to the inter-disciplinary nature of this research, I show how a number of theories influenced by argument. First, using the approaches used within the anthropology of development I provide a critique of HIV policymaking. Second, and in order to understand how policy was constructed based on misconceptions, I draw on elite and policymaking theories to demonstrate how the policy process is being mediated by the agendas of elites as opposed to bio-medical facts. Third, I use postcolonial theory to highlight how the elites are interpreting for themselves the colonial narrative that is founded on a binary opposition; civilised (the elites) and the uncivilised (the rural uneducated population) (Galtung 1971). This then enables the elites to distance themselves from those living in rural areas, allowing them to maintain a position of power and access to the resources flowing in from the aid community.

In this chapter I also review literature on HIV epidemiology. Epidemiological studies have estimated the risk of HIV-1 transmission. Although Malawians believe that HIV transmission is inevitable in a single act of unprotected intercourse (Anglewicz and Kohler 2009), epidemiologists found that the average rate of HIV transmission is 1 in 1000. These findings demonstrate that HIV is not easily transmitted. This is relevant to my study because the *fisi* practice occurs as a one-off heterosexual act and therefore it is statistically unlikely that this practice contributes significantly to the spread of HIV.

Moreover, the practice of *fisi* occurs in only a very small number of rural communities. In this chapter I also argue that the traditional practice of *fisi* is being utilised as a scapegoat for the spread of AIDS in Malawi to deliberately detract attention away from everyday sexual practices in urban areas of Malawi, such as extramarital relations and multiple sexual partners. As reflected in the evidence below, HIV prevalence is in fact higher in urban areas where the *fisi* practice does not take place.

In Chapter 3 I demonstrate the powerful and influential role that international donors (bilateral and multilateral agencies and INGOS) play in constructing AIDS policies and programmes. Additionally, this chapter emphasises that aid conditionality can fail to respond effectively to the AIDS epidemic by demonstrating how funding is often donor led. For example, if donors disagree with policies being implemented in the country to which they are supplying aid, whether it is the way money is being spent or the type of policies the government implements, then they will withdraw funds. I provide an example of the British Government suspending aid because it was unhappy with the President of Malawi's autocratic management style. The paradox of such policies in practice is that they reduce the ability of nation states to be self-sufficient and instead put them in a dependency relationship with international donors.

Data from the Malawi Demographic and Health Survey (2004) shows that urban residents have a significantly higher risk of HIV infection than rural residents. While 18% of urban women are HIV positive, the corresponding proportion for rural women is 13%. For men, the urban–rural difference in HIV prevalence is even greater; urban men are nearly twice as likely to be infected as rural men (16 and 9%, respectively) (MDHS 2004, p. 231). This is significant because harmful cultural practices are reported to be largely rural practices, yet infection rates are significantly higher in the urban areas where the majority of the elites—Malawians with at least a university education—live. This highlights the inaccuracy in the elites' narrative, one that blames rural Malawians for high prevalence rates. The problem is conversely higher in urban areas where the elites live. Further, HIV prevalence rates are higher among women aged 30–34 compared to women aged 15–19 (there is no data for women under 15). The fact that data was not collected and yet this is the demographic that is partaking in initiation ceremonies supports my argument that those blaming the sexual cultural practice of *fisi* for the spread of HIV lack evidence to support their case. In terms of education and wealth, the HIV prevalence rate is highest among women with a secondary education and above (15.1%) compared to those women with no education (13.6%). In terms of income those women with the highest rates of HIV were in the top wealth quintile. The emphasis of AIDS policies should therefore in fact be attributed more to contemporary patriarchal constructions of gender and power than a one-off highly un-evidenced traditional sexual practice.

I also examined how the advent of AIDS has provoked a reinterpretation of the impact of certain sexual cultural practices, which have now been labeled 'risky' or harmful. Some studies carried out have used culture as an explanation for high-risk behaviour, which can lead to HIV infection (Rushton and Bogaert 1989; Rushing 1995; Caldwell et al. 1989). However, this research shows that targeting specific population groups as opposed to addressing gender inequalities and issues of sexual power to a general population can be ineffective and misleading. This book does not argue that the cultural practices such as the *fisi* practice are not harmful and violent towards women but that these are not adversely contributing to the spread of HIV. Incorrect messages regarding HIV transmission rates are relayed which inhibit effective programme implementation.

Chapter 4 began by reviewing national and international policies on gender-based violence, harmful cultural practices and HIV/AIDS to highlight how these policies have been constructed around harmful cultural practices. I then reviewed literature on elites and used this to inform my own argument that policy processes are driven by elites as opposed to the argument made by Lasswell (1936) that policy implementation is a linear, rational process. These policies are being constructed around narratives of blame, which portray rural communities as backwards and the parties responsible for spreading HIV. This chapter concludes that the elites use these narratives as an 'imagined fact' in terms of how they contribute to high prevalence rates.

In Chapter 5 I argue that elite Christian religious morality has played an active role in portraying indigenous cultural practices as negative and blaming them for the spread of HIV/AIDS. In this chapter I also demonstrate how Christian elites portray themselves and their theology as enlightened in comparison to the minority Muslim population. Thus, casting indigenous cultural practices as responsible for the spread of AIDS with the agenda to undermine forms of traditional culture and validate a Christian lifestyle as unproblematic in terms of AIDS.

In Chapter 6 I examine theories of policy implementation, arguing against scholars such as Lasswell's (1936) presentation, that policy implementation is a linear, rational process. Instead, I agree with Lipsky (1980), Lindblom (1980), Shore and Wright (1997), and Sabatier (2007) who postulate that policy processes are less of a linear sequence but rather a political process underpinned by a complex mesh of interactions and ramifications between a wide range of stakeholders who are driven and constrained by competing interests and the context in which they operate.

I have argued that there are a wide range of stakeholders involved in policy construction and implementation. These stakeholders include large, and powerful bilateral and multilateral agencies, such as DFID, USAID and the World Bank, as well as international Non-governmental organisations, national NGOs, international and national faith-based organisations, and the organs of the Malawi government, both at the national and the district levels, each with its own vested interests and each with its own policies. Therefore I argue the evidence produced to apply policies is not objective evidence but narratives shaped by various policy agendas and interests of the elites. As a result policies are pushed in a direction that does not benefit the vast majority of Malawi's population in terms of HIV prevention, but instead perpetuate these groups' standings and beliefs.

THE THREE MAIN ARGUMENTS

In this book I argue that a complex interplay of interests has led to the construction of the narrative that the sexual cultural practice of *fisi* is contributing significantly to the spread of HIV and AIDS. I argue this interplay can be best understood through three sets of arguments. Although these three sets of arguments are presented separately here, in practice these are interlocking.

The first and main argument is that the 'narrative of blame' is maintained by the national elites in Malawi to ensure that HIV is kept on the development policy, thus attracting donor funding and retaining elites' professional status. I place emphasis on understanding policy construction as a process mediated by stakeholders involved in the policy process and argue that one reason why national elites are able to influence the policy agenda on HIV is due to the narrative they have constructed that has been sold to the donors. Thus they have a vested interest creating and maintaining the narrative of harmful cultural practices as responsible for the AIDS epidemic. This agenda permits them to maintain their own status and positions. Therefore, by maintaining the narrative that the sexual cultural practice of *fisi*, as well as other cultural practices that the elites consider harmful, drive the AIDS epidemic, they try to ensure that the policies and programmes directed to reduce HIV transmission continue.

The second argument identified in this study is that AIDS is presented by national, urban elites as a rural disease because the sexual cultural practice of *fisi* is reported to take place in rural areas. Therefore the narrative told by the elites is that the disease is being spread by people living in rural areas who are mainly illiterate and uncivilised. This narrative distances the urban elite from the disease, thus detracting attention from the higher level of AIDS in urban than in rural areas. As I highlight in this study, this 'othering' is a result of those elites working in HIV prevention providing explanations to 'problems' that satisfy donors and therefore ensure continued funding. Therefore, educated, urban elites who perceive themselves as civilised distance themselves from rural people who they position as uncivilised. I argue that elites in Malawi maintain their positions through adopting concepts of modernity held by the donors that rely upon a binary that divides the modern from the un-modern. Thus, the Malawian elites present themselves to donors, and potential donors, as suitable partners.

The third argument is that the Malawian elites have constructed a category of 'uncivilised', populated by those with little education (the majority of Malawians). They contrast these with themselves: educated Christians who are modern and progressive. This leads them to assert their superiority by placing the blame for the AIDS epidemic on those who practice what they call 'harmful cultural practices' that they associate with Malawian traditional religions. Within this context, Christian leaders play a role in projecting the narrative of blame as an ideological tool to promote a Christian lifestyle.

Contribution to AIDS Policy in Malawi

I have argued that although findings from epidemiological studies have shown that the probability of infection by one heterosexual act is 1 in 1000, I demonstrate that epidemiological evidence is ignored by policymakers. The gap between research and policy therefore needs to be bridged by disseminating research findings to policymakers so that when development programmes are designed they are based on evidence. Therefore for policy to be effective it needs to be informed by objective, empirical research on the population as a whole. For example, epidemiological evidence is particularly useful when preventing and controlling disease in populations and guiding health and health care policy and planning. Therefore such evidence can enrich health policies and plans to improve the health of a population.

The second contribution I make is a methodological one, enabling an understanding of how policy translates into practice across levels from the global arena down to the community level. The analytical framework and approach I proposed intended to facilitate analysis in evaluative and formative studies of—and policies and programmes on—AIDS, to generate meaningful evidence to inform policy. Therefore this study is not just applicable to Malawi but may be used in any country in the Global South. It is an original contribution to research as it focuses on narratives told by actors working in organisations, which focus on AIDS, while also tracing the impact of these narratives on the production of policies and programmes, rather than on geographically bounded local communities. My analytical framework has built on theoretical propositions and empirical research in development studies, particularly the work of Mosse (2011) and Crewe and Harrison (1998). I show that narratives on AIDS and sexual cultural practices are an obstacle to the development process. I argue these narratives become the dominant themes in the construction of policies. As a result, other key themes such as gendered power relationships are ignored or overlooked.

Thirdly, this study demonstrates a contribution to ethnographic research as it has shown how ethnography can be used to help construct policy and practice, which responds to the complexity of peoples' lives. Using this ethnographic approach has enabled me to highlight why progress is slow in terms of improving gender relations and has emphasised how these narratives of blame are used as a smokescreen to pursue government and donor interests.

The newspaper article by Nyasa Times 'Gender Minister wants women to hurt "hyenas"' tells the story of the Minister of Gender who, speaking at an event to commemorate 16 days of activism against gender-based violence, advised women to hurt the hyena. She is reported to have said 'Hit them (those hyenas) hard in their private parts and I can assure you it hurts' (*Nyasa Times* 2011). Of course, advising women to carry out violent acts towards men is not particularly helpful and will not help improve women's lives: to the contrary, it could leave them more vulnerable to abuse. But it is examples such as this one featured in the Malawi media that can be read by international donors and thereby influence international policy and programmes.

RECOMMENDATIONS

The following recommendations are based on the research I conducted for this study. What this research enabled me to do is develop my critical thinking on this issue.

- Policies and programmes developed on HIV/AIDS at the international and national level need to be informed by rigorous evidence, collected through critical, reflexive methodologies.
- To advance HIV/AIDS policies and programmes, stakeholders will need to embed policies in epidemiological evidence and pay greater

attention to how the wider political contexts at national and international levels impact on the policy and implementation processes.
- Stakeholders need to better articulate the link between sexual cultural practices, gender-based violence and women's health.
- Donors need to ensure they visit rural areas so that they understand the culture of the country and respond to local concerns and priorities.
- Quantification of the risk of HIV infection after sexual intercourse is difficult to measure therefore more quantitative studies are also needed regarding the risk of HIV infection after sexual intercourse to inform policy.
- Research needs to be accessible to non-academics. Researchers need to educate policymakers, by carrying out research that focuses on the ordinary cultural practices, such as extramarital relationships instead of the taken-for-granted understandings of rural people.

References

Anderson, E. L. (2012). Infectious women: Gendered bodies and HIV in Malawi. *International Feminist Journal of Politics, 14*(2), 267–287.
Anglewicz, P., & Kohler, H. P. (2009). Overestimating HIV infection: The construction and accuracy of subjective probabilities of HIV infection in rural Malawi. *Demography Research, 20*(6), 65–96.
Caldwell, J. C., Caldwell, P., & Quiggin, P. (1989). The social context of AIDS in sub-Saharan Africa. *Population and Development Review, 15*(2), 185–234.
Chimbiri, A. (2007). The condom is an 'intruder' in marriage: Evidence from rural Malawi. *Social Science and Medicine, 64*(5), 1102–1115.
Chin, J. (2007). *The AIDS pandemic: The collision of epidemiology with political correctness.* Oxford: Radcliffe Publishing.
Crewe, E., & Harrison, E. (1998). *Whose development? An ethnography of aid.* London: Zed.
Galtung, J. (1971). A structural theory of imperialism. *Journal of Peace Research, 8*(2), 81–117.
Gray, R. H., Wawer, M. J., Brookmeyer, R., Sewankambo, N. K., Serwadda, D., Wabwire-Mangen, F., ... & Quinn, T. C. (2001). Probability of HIV-1 transmission per coital act in monogamous, heterosexual, HIV-1-discordant couples in Rakai, Uganda. *The Lancet, 357*(9263), 1149–1153.
Kamlongera, A. (2007). What becomes of 'her'?: A look at the Malawian Fisi culture and its effects on young girls. *Agenda: Empowering Women for Gender Equity, 21*(74), 81–87.

Kistner, U., & Nkosi, Z. (2003). *Gender-based violence and HIV/AIDS in South Africa: A literature review.* Johannesburg: CADRE.
Lasswell, H. D. (1936). *Politics: Who gets what, when, how.* Cleveland: Meridian.
Lindblom, C. E. (1980). *The policy-making process.* Englewood Cliffs, NJ: Prentice Hall.
Lipsky, M. (1980). *Street-level bureaucracy: Dilemmas of the individual in public service.* New York: Russell Sage.
Malawi Demographic and Health Survey. (2004). Maryland: NSO and ORC Macro.
Mkamanga, E. (2000). *Suffering in silence-Malawi women's 30-year dance with Dr Banda.* Scotland: Dudu Nsomba Publications.
Mosse, D. (2011). Introduction: The anthropology of expertise and professionals in international development. In D. Mosse (Ed.), *Adventures in Aidland.* Oxford: Berghahn Books.
Nyasa Times. Retrieved November 29, 2011, from http://www.nyasatimes.com/2011/11/29/gender-minister-wants-women-to-hurt-hyenas/.
Packard, R. M., & Epstein, P. (1991). Epidemiologists, social scientists, and the structure of medical research on AIDS in Africa. *Social Science & Medicine, 33*(7), 771–794.
Powers, K. A., Poole, C., Pettifor, A. E., & Cohen, M. S. (2008). Rethinking the heterosexual infectivity of HIV-1: A systematic review and meta-analysis. *The Lancet Infectious Diseases, 8,* 553–563.
Rushing, W. A. (1995). *The AIDS epidemic: Social dimensions of an infectious disease.* Boulder, CO: Westview Press.
Rushton, J. P., & Bogaert, A. F. (1989). Population differences in susceptibility to AIDS: An evolutionary analysis. *Social Science & Medicine, 28*(12), 1211–1220.
Sabatier, P. A. (2007). The need for better theories. In P. Sabatier (Ed.), *Theories of the policy process.* Boulder, CO: Westview Press.
Shore, S., & Wright, S. (Eds.). (1997). *Anthropology of policy: Critical perspectives on governance and power.* London and New York: Routledge.
Waterston, A. (1997). Anthropological research and the politics of HIV prevention: Towards a critique of policy and priorities in the age of AIDS. *Social Science & Medicine, 44*(9), 1381–1391.

Open Access This chapter is licensed under the terms of the Creative Commons Attribution 4.0 International License (http://creativecommons.org/licenses/by/4.0/), which permits use, sharing, adaptation, distribution and reproduction in any medium or format, as long as you give appropriate credit to the original author(s) and the source, provide a link to the Creative Commons licence and indicate if changes were made.

The images or other third party material in this chapter are included in the chapter's Creative Commons licence, unless indicated otherwise in a credit line to the material. If material is not included in the chapter's Creative Commons licence and your intended use is not permitted by statutory regulation or exceeds the permitted use, you will need to obtain permission directly from the copyright holder.

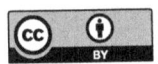

Glossary

Akunja	An outsider to the grace of the Christian God
Anankungwi	The traditional female initiation counsellor
Angaliba	The traditional male initiation counsellor among the Yao
Ankhoswe	The traditional marriage counsellor
Bwalo	Ground or open space in a village for meetings and *nyau* dances
Chiharo	The practice of widow inheritance: marrying the wife of a deceased brother
Chikule	The initial instruction given to a girl by her aunt or grandmother on her first menstruation
Chimwanamaye	Exchanging of husbands or wives
Chinamwali	Traditional initiation rite
Chisuweni	Female and male cousins are socially allowed to have sexual relationships
Chitayo	An illness believed to be caused by having sex during menstruation, soon after delivery or just after an abortion; also described as a hydrocele that develops in the scrotum of a man who has been in contact with a woman who is more than five months pregnant
Chokolo	The name of the widow herself in the practice of widow inheritance

Fisi	A man organised to have first sexual intercourse with a girl after commencement of menstruation or following initiation rite as symbol of maturity
Gwamula	Boys from different households sleep in one hut and invade a girls' hut; sometimes girls are forced to have sex with the boys
Jando/Mdulidwe	A male initiation ceremony that involves circumcision
Khundabwi	Herbal mixture given to a girl upon her first menstruation
Kuchotsa fumbi	Chichewa kulowa kufa (cleasing after death)
Kuchotsa milaza	Among the Chewa and Mang'anja, a widow may resume sexual intercourse without the disturbance of the spouse's spirit in her after experiencing sexual cleansing with the deceased's relative, thereby re-entering the life cycle
Kulowa kufa	Cleansing after death
Kupita kufa	Sexual cleansing involving the surviving spouse with a relative from the other side of the family; it can take place for men or women
Kusasa fumbi	Sexual intercourse done soon after undergoing initiation rituals
Kutenga mwana	Newborn cleansing
Matrilocal	Upon marriage, the husband relocates to the local group of the wife, generally to her mother's household compound
Matripotestal	Authority over the members of the family is in the hands of the mother or relatives
Mbulo	Temporary husband replacement
M'bvade	Where an unmarried female's post-natal abstinence is concluded by surrogate sex
Mdulo	Mysterious disease caused by the transgression of a sexual taboo
Mitala	Polygamy
Mkangali	The last stage of a chief's initiation rite
Mphini	Ear piercing and tattooing,
Mwambo	Custom
Nkhoswe	A go-between to handle marriage negotiations and marriage affairs

Nthena	Widow cleansing: in the Northern region, where a widower is given a wife's younger sister
Nyau cult	The Chewa secret male society
Patrilocal	Upon marriage, the wife relocates to the local group of the husband, generally to her father-in-law's household compound
Polygyny	Having multiple wives
Tsempho	An illness that appears like AIDS

INDEX

A
Actors, 144–146, 150, 151, 156, 157, 159–161
Aid, 44–49, 57
Aid community, 38
Aid conditionality, 49, 57
Aid game in Malawi, 141
 the aid game, 141
AIDS, 2–19, 61, 65–67, 69–73, 75, 76, 80, 81, 84, 88, 91, 92, 99, 101, 103, 141–144, 147, 155, 157, 159, 160, 162–164, 166–171, 173–175
 HIV, 2, 4–8, 10, 11, 13–19
 HIV prevalence rates, 7, 11
AIDS exceptionalism, 50
AIDS policies and programmes, 47, 49, 50, 57
Anthropology of development, 25, 38

B
Biomedical evidence, 143, 145, 166

C
Christianity, 107–109, 114, 117, 135
Church, 107, 111–114, 116–120, 124, 125, 129, 130, 133–135
Civilised and uncivilised, 38
Colonial narrative, 38
Conclusion, 187, 188
Cultural practices, 109, 114, 117–126, 129, 130, 133, 136, 144, 151, 154, 155, 157, 159, 160, 163–171, 173–175
 cultural practices as harmful, 129, 130, 136
 sexual cultural practices, 114, 136
Culture, 55, 56
 cultural norms, 54
 societal norms, 55
Customs and practices, 71, 72

D
Development aid situation, 43
Development buzzwords, 126, 129
Development issues, 70

Development policy process, 145
Donor interest, 112
donor interest and funding of religious groups in development, 112
Donor led funding, 49, 57
Donors, 146–148, 154–156, 159, 160, 162–164, 168, 170, 173
Donors influencing policy process, 74
Donors (role of), 4–6, 9–11, 14, 15, 18, 19

E
Education, 1, 2, 5, 10, 12, 13, 18
Elites, 4–10, 12, 14, 17, 18
Elite theory, elites, 26, 27, 33
Enlightenment, 134
Epidemiology, epidemiology of HIV, 35, 37, 38
Epidemiology of virus, 103
Epistemic community, 5, 14, 15
Ethnographic research, 195
ethnography of aid, 8
Evidence, 4–8, 15, 142–144, 146–148, 155, 160, 161, 163, 164, 166–168, 170, 175, 176, 180
  anthropological evidence, 7
  epidemiological evidence, 6, 7
Evidence-based policy, 188

F
Findings, 187, 188, 190, 194
  summary of findings, 189
fisi (hyena), 2, 7, 8, 10, 13, 18

G
Gender-based violence, 188, 192, 195

H
Harmful cultural practices, 2, 4, 5, 12, 14, 16, 18, 61, 62, 65–67, 69, 79, 84, 89, 90, 92, 103, 104
  exotic cultural practices, 6
  sexual cultural practices, 5, 18
HIV epidemiology, 189, 190
HIV prevention, 65, 88, 100, 104, 141–143, 145, 167, 174, 180
HIV infection, 142
HIV transmission, 142, 174

I
Initiation rites, 130–134
International donors, 187, 190, 191, 195
International donors (bilateral and multilateral agencies and INGOS), 47, 49, 57
International frameworks, 67, 80
International frameworks and agendas, 28
Interviews, 84, 91, 92, 103, 141, 144, 147, 166

M
Malawi, 1–16, 18, 19, 43–45, 47–55, 57
  Malawi´s national HIV policy, 51
Malawian elite, 80, 84, 90, 103, 129, 187, 189, 194
  Chirsitian religious elites, 136
  national and district elites, 81
  religious elite, 136
Misconceptions, 25, 38
Modernity, 136
Multiple sexual partners, 55, 56

N

Narratives, 141, 144, 146, 147, 151, 157, 158, 160, 161, 164, 173, 180
  narratives shaped by various policy agendas and interests of the elites, 193
Narratives of blame, 18, 192, 195
Neo liberalism, 44, 45
Networks, 145, 151, 157, 159, 161
Non-Governmental Organisation (NGO), 1, 2, 4–7, 9–12, 14

P

Patriarchy, 54
Policy, 25–28, 30, 32–34, 37, 38, 62–67, 70, 77, 81, 88, 92
  global policies, 62, 66
  policies and programmes, 25, 28
  policy making, 26, 27, 32, 33, 38
Policy construction, 141
Post-colonial theory, 29
Power, 25–28, 30–32, 36, 38
Probability of infection, 188, 194

R

Recommendations, 187, 189, 195
Religion, 107–109, 112, 115, 116, 130, 132
  religion and AIDS, 112
Rural people, 103
  rural communities, 103

S

Schools of policy making, 148
Sexual behaviour, 187
Sexual cultural practices, 187, 191, 195, 196
Stakeholders, 141, 144, 146, 161, 162, 168, 176
Sub Saharan Africa, 28

T

Theories of policy implementation, 148
Theories, theoretical perspectives, 25
  theoretical framework, 25
Traditional practices, 61–63, 65, 68, 104
  cultural practices, 62, 68

U

Uneducated and backward farmers, 136

V

Violence, 187, 188, 196
Violence against women, 61, 62, 65, 66
  gender based violence, 66

Y

Young women and girls, 11

The manufacturer's authorised representative in the EU is Springer Nature Customer Service Centre GmbH, Europaplatz 3, 69115 Heidelberg, Germany. If you have any concerns regarding our products, please contact ProductSafety@springernature.com

Printed and bound by CPI Group (UK) Ltd, Croydon, CR0 4YY
23/03/2026
02076667-0001